Inflammatory Bowel Disease

An Evidence-based Practical Guide

Edited by
Ailsa L Hart
Siew C Ng

tfm Publishing Limited, Castle Hill Barns, Harley, Nr Shrewsbury, SY5 6LX, UK
Tel: +44 (0)1952 510061; Fax: +44 (0)1952 510192
E-mail: nikki@tfmpublishing.com;
Web site: www.tfmpublishing.com

Design & Typesetting: Nikki Bramhill BSc Hons Dip Law
First Edition: © 2012
ISBN: 978 1 903378 82 3

Printed by Gutenberg Press Ltd.,
Gudja Road, Tarxien, PLA 19, Malta
Tel: +356 21897037; Fax: +356 21800069

Contents

Part 3

Contributors

Ayesha Akbar MRCP PhD Consultant Gastroenterologist, St Mark's Hospital, London, UK

Lachlan R. O. Ayres MBChB MRCP(UK) Gastroenterology and General (Internal) Medicine Specialty Registrar, Bristol Royal Infirmary, Bristol, UK

Gareth Bashir MEd FRCS Surgical Registrar, St Mark's Hospital, London, UK

Paul A. Blaker BSc MBBS MRCP Research Fellow in Gastroenterology, Guy's & St Thomas' Hospital, London, UK

Helen Campbell BSc SRD Dietitian, Guy's & St Thomas' NHS Foundation Trust, London, UK

Nishchay Chandra MRCP Consultant Gastroenterologist, Department of Gastroenterology, Royal Berkshire Hospital, Reading, UK

Susan K. Clark MA MB BChir MD FRCS(Gen Surg) Consultant Colorectal Surgeon, St Mark's Hospital, London, UK

J. R. Fraser Cummings FRCP DPhil Consultant Gastroenterologist, Department of Gastroenterology, University Hospital Southampton, Southampton, UK

Edward J. Despott MD MRCP(UK) Advanced Endoscopy Research Fellow, Wolfson Unit for Endoscopy, St Mark's Hospital and Academic Institute, Imperial College London, UK

John M. E. Fell MA MD MRCP FRCPCH Consultant Paediatric Gastroenterologist, Chelsea and Westminster Hospital, London, UK

Chris Fraser MB ChB MD FRCP Consultant Gastroenterologist and Specialist Endoscopist, Wolfson Unit for Endoscopy, St Mark's Hospital and Academic Institute; Honorary Senior Lecturer, Imperial College London, UK

Simon M. Gabe MD MSc BSc MBBS FRCP Consultant Gastroenterologist, St Mark's Hospital, London, UK

Ailsa L. Hart BMBCh MRCP PhD Senior Clinical Lecturer, Imperial College and Consultant Gastroenterologist, St Mark's Hospital, London, UK

Gwo-Tzer Ho MRCP PhD Consultant Gastroenterologist and MRC Clinician Scientist, University of Edinburgh, Western General Hospital, Edinburgh, Scotland

Peter M. Irving MA MD MRCP Consultant Gastroenterologist, Guy's & St Thomas' Hospital, London, UK

Satish Keshav MBBCh DPhil FRCP Consultant Gastroenterologist and Honorary Senior Lecturer, Translational Gastroenterology Unit, John Radcliffe Hospital and University of Oxford, Oxford, UK

Jonathan Landy MRCP Research Fellow and Specialist Registrar, St Mark's Hospital, London, UK

James Lindsay PhD BM BCh FRCP Senior Lecturer, Barts and the London School of Medicine and Dentistry, Queen Mary University of London; Consultant Gastroenterologist, Barts and the London NHS Trust, London, UK

Craig Mowat MD FRCP Consultant Gastroenterologist, Ninewells Hospital and Medical School, Dundee, Scotland

Siew Ng MBBS PhD MRCP Assistant Professor, Institute of Digestive Disease, Department of Medicine and Therapeutics, Chinese University of Hong Kong, Hong Kong; Senior Lecturer and Honorary Gastroenterologist, St Vincent's Hospital, University of Melbourne, Australia

Jeremy Nightingale MB BS FRCP MD Cert MHS Consultant in Gastroenterology and Nutritional Support, St Mark's Hospital, London, UK

Timothy R. Orchard MA MD DM FHEA FRCP Consultant Gastroenterologist, Imperial College Healthcare Trust and Reader in Gastroenterology, Imperial College London, St Mary's Hospital, London, UK

Simon Peake MRCP Research Fellow and Specialist Registrar, St Mark's Hospital, London, UK

Charlotte Pither BSc (Hons) BM MRCP Specialist Registrar, Department of Gastroenterology, University Hospital Southampton, Southampton, UK

Sophie Plamondon MD FRCPC Assistant Professor of Medicine, Université de Sherbrooke, Faculty of Medicine, Division of Gastroenterology, Centre Hospitalier Universitaire de Sherbrooke, Québec, Canada; Centre de Recherche Étienne-LeBel, Québec, Canada

Chris S. J. Probert MD FRCP FHEA Professor of Gastroenterology, University of Bristol, School of Clinical Science, Bristol Royal Infirmary, Bristol, UK

Jean-François Rahier MD Service d'Hépatogastroentérologie, Cliniques Universitaires UCL Mont-Godinne, Yvoir, Belgium

Joannie Ruel MD Assistant Professor of Medicine, Université de Sherbrooke, Faculty of Medicine, Division of Gastroenterology, Centre Hospitalier Universitaire de Sherbrooke, Québec, Canada

Evangelos A. Russo MBBS MRCP Clinical Research Fellow and Honorary Specialist Registrar in Gastroenterology, Imperial College London, Clinical Imaging Centre, Hammersmith Hospital, London, UK

Jeremy Sanderson MD FRCP Consultant Gastroenterologist, Guy's & St. Thomas' NHS Foundation Trust; Reader in Gastroenterology, Department of Nutrition, King's College London, UK

Brian P. Saunders MD FRCP Consultant Gastroenterologist, Wolfson Unit for Endoscopy, St Mark's Hospital, London, UK

Stephen Tattersall MBBS FRACP Consultant Gastroenterologist, Concord Hospital, Australia

Kirstin M. Taylor BSc MRCP Clinical Research Fellow, Guy's & St Thomas' NHS Foundation Trust & King's College London, UK

Cheng T. Tee MB BCh BAO MRCP(UK)(Gastroenterology) Research Fellow, St Mark's Hospital, London, UK

Siwan Thomas-Gibson MD FRCP Consultant Gastroenterologist, Wolfson Unit for Endoscopy, St Mark's Hospital, London, UK

Phil Tozer MBBS MRCS Eng MCEM Research Fellow, St Mark's Hospital, London, UK; Imperial College London, UK

Carolynne Vaizey MBChB MD FRCS(Gen) FCS(SA) Consultant Colorectal Surgeon, St Mark's Hospital, London, UK

Janindra Warusavitarne BMed PhD FRACS Consultant Colorectal Surgeon, St Mark's Hospital, London, UK

Josef Watfah MD Surgical Registrar, St Mark's Hospital, London, UK

Foreword

The pace of change in the management of inflammatory bowel disease (IBD) has accelerated over the past decade. It is an exciting time for physicians, surgeons and nurse specialists caring for patients with IBD. As our clinical experience and trial data accumulate, several important lessons have been learnt, and there is now a need for a practical guide as to how best to use currently available drugs when managing patients in our clinical practice. Our vision was to provide a book with succinct chapters illustrating therapeutic pathways and algorithms of care to achieve best outcomes for patients in day-to-day practice. This book is suitable for all medical professionals involved in the care of patients with IBD, established and trainee gastroenterologists, gastrointestinal surgeons, nurse specialists, general practitioners and general physicians across the globe.

Inflammatory Bowel Disease – An Evidence-based Practical Guide is a collection of evidence and experience from renowned IBD physicians and surgeons highlighting evidence for existing and new therapies in IBD supported by logical therapeutic pathways. It is characterised by the management of simple and complex Crohn's disease and ulcerative colitis as well as special scenarios pertaining to the management of extra-intestinal manifestations, optimal colorectal cancer surveillance, best use of drugs during pregnancy and breast feeding, and how and when to screen for infections.

We were fortunate to receive excellent training in IBD in the same institute, St Mark's Hospital, London and under the same mentor, Professor Michael Kamm, whose vision is an inspiration. The opportunity to work together on this book was a unique one – an idea that fertilised during a plane flight, and chapters that flourished through several Skype conversations. Although we now practise across the continents, we not only enjoy each other's encouragement and stimulating ideas, but also share the same passion in advancing and pioneering practice for IBD. We are extremely grateful to the authors of the chapters, who are internationally renowned physicians and surgeons, and excellent colleagues.

This endeavour would not have been possible without our publisher Nikki Bramhill (Director, tfm publishing Ltd). It has been a real pleasure and delight to work with Nikki and share stories of our 'little ones' whilst of course working hard on the book.

Ailsa L. Hart and Siew C. Ng

Dedications

Dedication for this book goes to my family and Graham for unconditional support and to my beautiful one-year-old daughter, Olivia, who never fails to make every day a special one.

SCN

Dedication goes to my wonderful family, Andy, Ollie, Edward and my parents, who mean the world to me – where would I be without their love and support.

ALH

Part 1 Introduction

Management of ulcerative colitis

Ailsa L. Hart BMBCh MRCP PhD Senior Clinical Lecturer, Imperial College and Consultant Gastroenterologist, St Mark's Hospital, London, UK

Ulcerative colitis is an inflammatory bowel disease of unknown cause (idiopathic) that affects up to 120,000 people in the UK with between 6,000 and 12,000 new cases being diagnosed each year.

The principal symptoms of ulcerative colitis include diarrhoea with rectal bleeding, abdominal pain and cramps, usually relieved by defecation. Symptoms depend on the extent and severity of disease. When disease extends beyond the rectum, patients tend to complain of diarrhoea (often with blood and mucus), faecal urgency and faecal incontinence. Patients with disease limited to the rectum (proctitis) tend to present with rectal bleeding and mucus discharge and a proportion of these patients complain of constipation, as opposed to diarrhoea. Patients with a more severe colitis have associated systemic symptoms of fever, vomiting and anorexia. One way of classifying ulcerative colitis is using the Montreal classification (Table 1) which takes into account the part of the colon affected [1].

Table 1. Montreal classification of ulcerative colitis.

E1	Limited to rectum
E2	Colorectum distal to splenic flexure
E3	Involvement extends proximal to splenic flexure

Ulcerative colitis tends to begin in the rectum and extends proximally affecting the bowel in a continuous fashion. Approximately one third of patients have disease confined to the rectum (proctitis) or the rectum and sigmoid (proctosigmoiditis) at the time of diagnosis. Approximately one third of patients will have a pancolitis at diagnosis. Disease can progress and extend, so that patients who have rectal or rectosigmoid involvement at presentation can progress to have disease affecting the proximal colon in 10-30% of patients at 10-year follow-up and in up to 50% at 25-year follow-up [2, 3].

The pattern of disease can follow different courses. Most patients have a chronic intermittent course with periods of remission and relapse [3]; a cumulative relapse rate in the first year after diagnosis is about 50% irrespective of disease extent. Other patients have chronic continuous symptoms. Some patients have a single attack and subsequent remission. Some patients have a fulminant course leading to colectomy within the first disease episode. About 10% of patients have long-term remission after the initial disease episode. The extent of disease at diagnosis does not seem to affect the subsequent disease activity. When patients are followed up long term, disease activity in the previous year appears to be a good indicator of the subsequent course of disease [3]. For example, a full year in remission is prognostically favourable and predicts an 80% probability of staying in remission for another year. The more years in remission, the higher the probability of experiencing yet another year in remission. On the other hand relapse in the previous year predicts a 70% probability of relapse in the subsequent year.

Both disease activity and extent determine treatment choice in the management of ulcerative colitis. For this reason this section is divided into chapters in which the extent of disease (e.g. proctitis, left-sided disease, extensive disease) and severity of disease (e.g. acute severe ulcerative colitis) are taken into account.

Each chapter has an algorithm of care, but in practice the care is individualised to the patient. Factors that contribute to the individual management of patients include patient preferences and beliefs; external factors such as schooling, work and family lives that may influence timing and choice of certain treatments; intolerance to medications; and other comorbidities. A clear agenda with a time-bound approach needs to be discussed with the patient, so that expectations of both the patient and health care professionals can be explored and met.

Treatment goals in ulcerative colitis include induction and maintenance of remission, mucosal healing, avoidance of admission to hospital, avoidance of surgery, minimising the risk of cancer, and optimised quality of life. Definition of remission and the contribution of clinical aspects, endoscopy, biomarkers and histopathology remain to be decided, but the bar should be raised with regards to what patients and physicians aim to achieve. An improvement in symptoms and wellbeing is unlikely to predict long-term outcome and is no longer optimal.

Treatment options for ulcerative colitis are increasing with development of new drug formulations and dosing strategies. There is a greater appreciation that assessment needs to occur in a timely fashion so that therapy can be escalated and optimised. There is also increased awareness of compliance problems that may need to be discussed and addressed.

References

1. Silverberg MS, Satsangi J, Ahmad T, *et al.* Toward an integrated clinical, molecular and serological classification of inflammatory bowel disease: Report of a Working Party of the 2005 Montreal World Congress of Gastroenterology. *Can J Gastroenterol* 2005; 19 Suppl A: 5-36.
2. Ayres RC, Gillen CD, Walmsley RS, Allan RN. Progression of ulcerative proctosigmoiditis: incidence and factors influencing progression. *Eur J Gastroenterol Hepatol* 1996; 8: 555-8.
3. Langholz E, Munkholm P, Davidsen M, Binder V. Course of ulcerative colitis: analysis of changes in disease activity over years. *Gastroenterology* 1994; 107: 3-11.

Chapter 1

Management of ulcerative proctitis

Siew Ng MBBS PhD MRCP Assistant Professor, Institute of Digestive Disease, Department of Medicine and Therapeutics, Chinese University of Hong Kong, Hong Kong; Senior Lecturer and Honorary Gastroenterologist, St Vincent's Hospital, University of Melbourne, Australia

Overview

Ulcerative proctitis is defined as inflammation that is limited to the rectum. Symptoms include rectal bleeding, urgency and tenesmus. Diagnosis can be confirmed by symptom assessment and sigmoidoscopy. Epidemiological studies have shown that proctitis represents 25-55% of ulcerative colitis. Topical 5-aminosalicylate (5-ASA) is superior to oral 5-ASA or topical steroids, and is the first-line treatment of choice to induce remission. Long-term follow-up studies suggest that topical 5-ASA is better than placebo to maintain remission. In patients who do not respond to topical 5-ASA or steroids, the addition of oral 5-ASA, immunosuppressants and anti-tumour necrosis factor agents may be effective. Cyclosporine, tacrolimus or arsenic suppositories can be considered in resistant cases. Surgery is rarely needed.

Introduction

Proctitis, or E1 by the Montreal classification, is disease localised to the rectum. It occurs in up to 50% of patients with ulcerative colitis at diagnosis. Although proctitis is associated with symptoms of increasing stool frequency, rectal bleeding, tenesmus and urgency, it can often be managed in the community. Treatment guidelines recommend endoscopy and symptom assessment to confirm the diagnosis of ulcerative colitis and to determine the extent and severity of the disease. The goal of therapy is to induce remission and to maintain long-term remission and improvement in quality of life. Topical medication with 5-aminosalicylic acid (5-ASA) is effective and considered first-line therapy in most patients with proctitis. Topical 5-ASA is more efficacious than oral compounds. The combination of topical 5-ASA and oral 5-ASA or topical steroids should be considered for escalation of treatment in those with suboptimal response. For the maintenance of remission, 5-ASA suppositories are used if acceptable by patients, although in clinical practice this depends on the patient's level of education and preference. Some patients may prefer oral 5-ASA as maintenance therapy which might prevent proximal extension of the disease. Resistant proctitis can be challenging to manage. Physicians should have a low threshold to perform a flexible sigmoidoscopy to assess the extent of disease in patients not responding, to allow targeted therapy according to the location of residual inflammation. In patients with chronically active proctitis refractory or intolerant to topical 5-ASAs and corticosteroids, immunomodulators or biological therapy is an alternative option. Other novel agents including tacrolimus, cyclosporine or arsenic suppositories can be considered prior to proctocolectomy.

Population-based studies have shown that the incidence of colorectal cancer in patients with limited disease is low [1, 2]; therefore, the European consensus guideline and international expert opinion suggest that patients with proctitis do not require surveillance.

Topical 5-ASA

Topical 5-ASA therapy is the most effective first-line treatment in patients with proctitis. Suppositories can reach the upper rectum (15-

20cm proximal to the anal verge), whereas enemas may reach the splenic flexure although they rarely concentrate in the rectum. In patients with proctitis, a 1g Pentasa suppository daily induced faster clinical and endoscopic remission, and was better tolerated, than a 500mg suppository twice daily [3, 4]. A recent study showed that once-daily administration of a 1g mesalamine (Salofalk) suppository is as effective and safe as the standard thrice-daily administration of a 500mg mesalamine suppository. Remission rates were 87.9% and 90.7%, respectively [5]. Topical 5-ASA also induced earlier and better remission rates than oral 5-ASA in patients with active proctitis [6-8]. This may relate to a decreased exposure of the distal colon to orally-dosed topical agents because of asymmentric distribution of 5-ASA within the colon. 5-ASA primarily exerts therapeutic effects at a mucosal level and high topical concentrations of 5-ASA delivered to the sites of inflammation is crucial for optimal efficacy. Topical 5-ASA also plays an important role in maintaining remission in proctitis [9, 10], although due to patient preference oral agents are often used as an alternative.

If once-daily 5-ASA suppositories at night fail to induce a response, the frequency of suppositories can be increased to two to three times over 24 hours to provide constant mucosal exposure, which is sometimes effective in inducing remission. The 3- or 4-hour morning period of increased bowel frequency is best avoided, but by late morning the use of suppositories can be resumed. However, this strategy has not been assessed in a controlled manner. Once remission is achieved patients can be maintained with alternate day 5-ASA suppository or daily oral 5-ASA.

Topical steroids

Prednisolone-21-phosphate suppositories have been shown to be an effective therapy for patients with idiopathic proctitis [11, 12]. Alternative glucocorticoids such as budesonide and beclometasone dipropionate are also available in suppository form or enemas. An early study comparing the efficacy and tolerance of 5-ASA suppositories and hydrocortisone acetate foam showed that although both treatments reduced disease activity in acute proctitis, 5-ASA suppositories were more effective than hydrocortisone in reducing rectal blood loss, mucus discharge and endoscopy score [13]. Overall, topical 5-ASA is at least twice as effective as topical steroids for symptom improvement, endoscopic remission and histological improvement. Rectal steroids are not recommended as maintenance therapy for proctitis due to the lack of long-term maintenance data and the risk of cumulative systemic absorption [14].

Management of resistant proctitis

Few studies have evaluated therapies for refractory proctitis. If rectal 5-ASA or corticosteroid therapy is ineffective, poor compliance to therapy, superimposed infection and proximal disease extension should be considered. A combination of oral corticosteroids with rectal 5-ASA can be considered in patients refractory to monotherapy. Chronically active patients refractory to, or intolerant of, rectal and oral 5-ASAs and corticosteroids require immunomodulators (azathioprine or 6-MP) or biological therapy, although evidence for the latter is limited [15]. In a recent study, infliximab therapy induced and maintained remission in patients with resistant proctitis. Nine of 13 patients (69%) had a complete response, 2/13 (15%) had a partial response and 2/13 (15%) did not respond at a median follow-up of 17 months. Among the 11 patients with clinical response after infliximab induction therapy, 9 (82%) patients maintained response at last follow-up. Endoscopic mucosal improvement was seen in seven patients. One patient underwent proctocolectomy [16].

Other novel therapies

More experimental therapies such as nicotine enemas and patches, short-chain fatty acid enemas [17], arsenic (acetarsol) suppositories [18], cyclosporine enemas [19, 20] and epidermal growth factor enemas can be considered in resistant proctitis [21, 22].

Although the use of arsenic suppositories for the treatment of resistant proctitis was first described in 1965 [12], there has since been only one small open-label study reporting the use of acetarsol suppositories 250mg twice daily for 4 weeks in ten patients. Nine of ten patients achieved symptomatic and endoscopic improvement within 2 weeks. Side effects were minimal and arsenic levels fell rapidly when acetarsol was withdrawn.

Short-term acetarsol therapy appeared to be a useful and safe measure in resistant proctitis [18].

Two prospective studies have demonstrated the efficacy of rectal tacrolimus (tacrolimus suppository or enema) in patients with distal colitis resistant to standard and experimental therapies. In one study of eight patients with proctitis (maximum 30cm inflammation from anus) refractory to 5-ASA, steroids, immunosuppressants and infliximab, six of eight patients achieved clinical remission [23]. A separate study showed that 13 of 19 patients with distal colitis responded to 4 weeks of rectal tacrolimus, with no major side effects [24]. Further controlled studies are now warranted.

Appendectomy may have a role in the treatment of proctitis. In a prospective case series study, 30 adult patients with ulcerative proctitis underwent appendicectomy in the absence of any history suggestive of previous appendicitis. Twenty-seven of 30 (90%) patients achieved clinical improvement and 12 of 30 (40%) patients had clinical remission at 12 months [25]. In a case series of eight patients with proctitis refractory to treatment with mesalazine orally and topically, elective appendicectomy resulted in mucosal healing of proctitis in all patients with follow-up of 3.6 years. A controlled study is currently in progress [26].

A treatment algorithm for the management of proctitis is outlined in Figure 1.

Conclusions

Ulcerative proctitis can be challenging to manage. The first-line therapy is topical 5-ASAs. In patients who do not respond to rectal 5-ASA suppositories 1g daily, increasing the frequency of rectal therapy to two to three suppositories per day may be effective. Failing that, the addition of topical steroid therapy (prednisolone-21-phosphate suppositories), oral 5-ASA or oral steroids should be used. Chronically active patients refractory to combined rectal and oral treatment will require azathioprine, 6-MP or infliximab. Prior to the consideration of surgery, acetarsol suppositories or cyclosporine/tacrolimus enemas may enable some patients to achieve remission although data have been based on uncontrolled data.

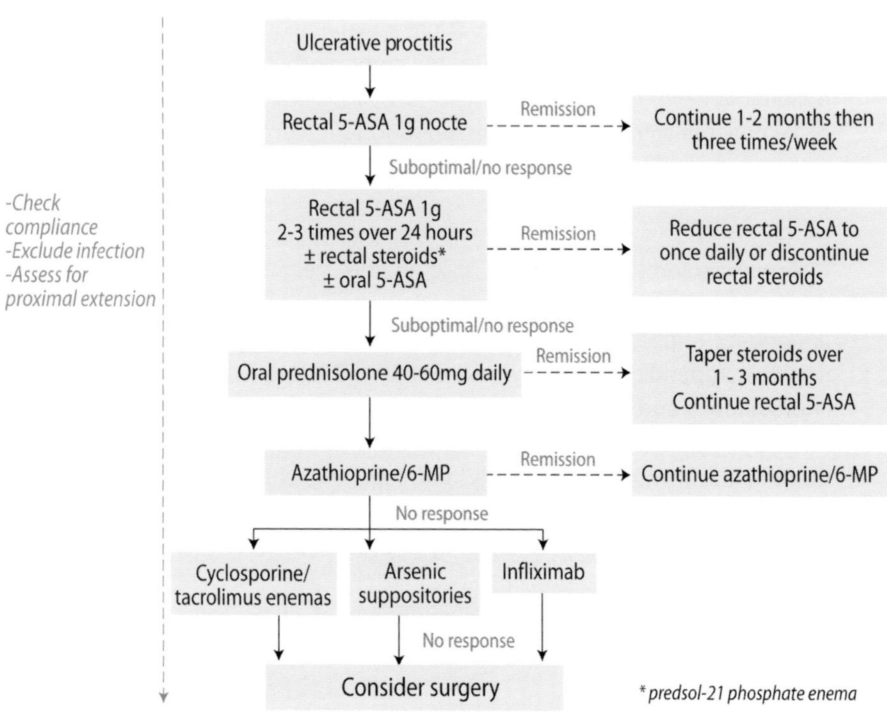
-Check compliance
-Exclude infection
-Assess for proximal extension
Ulcerative proctitis
Rectal 5-ASA 1g nocte
Remission
Continue 1-2 months then three times/week
Suboptimal/no response
Rectal 5-ASA 1g
2-3 times over 24 hours
± rectal steroids*
± oral 5-ASA
Remission
Reduce rectal 5-ASA to once daily or discontinue rectal steroids
Suboptimal/no response
Oral prednisolone 40-60mg daily
Remission
Taper steroids over
1 - 3 months
Continue rectal 5-ASA
Azathioprine/6-MP
Remission
Continue azathioprine/6-MP
No response
Cyclosporine/
tacrolimus enemas
Arsenic
suppositories
Infliximab
No response
Consider surgery
* predsol-21 phosphate enema

Figure 1. Treatment algorithm for the management of proctitis.

Key points

- Topical 5-ASA is more effective than topical steroids to induce and maintain remission in proctitis.
- The addition of oral 5-ASA or topical steroids is beneficial if topical 5-ASA alone is ineffective or poorly tolerated.
- Poor compliance to therapy, superimposed infection and proximal disease extension should be considered in patients who fail to respond to topical 5-ASA.
- Refractory proctitis may benefit from the addition of thiopurine, anti-TNF, tacrolimus/cyclosporine enemas or arsenic suppositories; the risk and efficacy of each approach should be addressed in individual patients.

References

1. Ekbom A, Helmick C, Zack M, *et al.* Ulcerative colitis and colorectal cancer. A population-based study. *N Engl J Med* 1990; 323: 1228-33.
2. Heuschen UA, Hinz U, Allemeyer EH, *et al.* Backwash ileitis is strongly associated with colorectal carcinoma in ulcerative colitis. *Gastroenterology* 2001; 120: 841-7.
3. Gionchetti P, Rizzello F, Venturi A, *et al.* Comparison of mesalazine suppositories in proctitis and distal proctosigmoiditis. *Aliment Pharmacol Ther* 1997; 11: 1053-7.
4. Marteau P, Florent C. Comparative, open, randomized trial of the efficacy and tolerance of slow-release 5-ASA suppositories once daily versus conventional 5-ASA suppositories twice daily in the treatment of active cryptogenic proctitis: French Pentasa Study Group. *Am J Gastroenterol* 2000; 95: 166-70.
5. Andus T, Kocjan A, Muser M, *et al.* Clinical trial: a novel high-dose 1g mesalamine suppository (Salofalk) once daily is as efficacious as a 500mg suppository thrice daily in active ulcerative proctitis. *Inflamm Bowel Dis* 2010; 16: 1947-56.
6. Gionchetti P, Rizzello F, Venturi A, *et al.* Comparison of oral with rectal mesalazine in the treatment of ulcerative proctitis. *Dis Colon Rectum* 1998; 41: 93-7.
7. Safdi M, DeMicco M, Sninsky C, *et al.* A double-blind comparison of oral versus rectal mesalamine versus combination therapy in the treatment of distal ulcerative colitis. *Am J Gastroenterol* 1997; 92: 1867-71.
8. Kam L, Cohen H, Dooley C, *et al.* A comparison of mesalamine suspension enema and oral sulfasalazine for treatment of active distal ulcerative colitis in adults. *Am J Gastroenterol* 1996; 91: 1338-42.

9. Regueiro MD. Diagnosis and treatment of ulcerative proctitis. *J Clin Gastroenterol* 2004; 38: 733-40.
10. Regueiro M, Loftus EV, Jr., Steinhart AH, *et al.* Medical management of left-sided ulcerative colitis and ulcerative proctitis: critical evaluation of therapeutic trials. *Inflamm Bowel Dis* 2006; 12: 979-94.
11. Lennard-Jones JE, Baron JH, Connell AM, *et al.* A double blind controlled trial of prednisolone-21-phosphate suppositories in the treatment of idiopathic proctitis. *Gut* 1962; 3: 207-10.
12. Connell AM, Lennard-Jones JE, Misiewicz JJ, *et al.* Comparison of acetarsol and prednisolone-21-phosphate suppositories in the treatment of idiopathic proctitis. *Lancet* 1965; 1: 238.
13. Lucidarme D, Marteau P, Foucault M, *et al.* Efficacy and tolerance of mesalazine suppositories vs. hydrocortisone foam in proctitis. *Aliment Pharmacol Ther* 1997; 11: 335-40.
14. Luboshitzky R, Rachelis Z, Nussensone E, *et al.* Beclomethasone dipropionate enema in ulcerative colitis: is it safe? *Endocr Pract* 2009; Jun 2: 1-18.
15. Lakatos PL, Lakatos L. Ulcerative proctitis: a review of pharmacotherapy and management. *Expert Opin Pharmacother* 2008; 9: 741-9.
16. Bouguen G, Roblin X, Bourreille A, *et al.* Infliximab for refractory ulcerative proctitis. *Aliment Pharmacol Ther* 2010; 31: 1178-85.
17. Pinto A, Fidalgo P, Cravo M, *et al.* Short chain fatty acids are effective in short-term treatment of chronic radiation proctitis: randomized, double-blind, controlled trial. *Dis Colon Rectum* 1999; 42: 788-95.
18. Forbes A, Britton TC, House IM, *et al.* Safety and efficacy of acetarsol suppositories in unresponsive proctitis. *Aliment Pharmacol Ther* 1989; 3: 553-6.
19. Ranzi T, Campanini MC, Velio P, *et al.* Treatment of chronic proctosigmoiditis with cyclosporin enemas. *Lancet* 1989; 2: 97.
20. Brynskov J, Freund L, Thomsen OO, *et al.* Treatment of refractory ulcerative colitis with cyclosporin enemas. *Lancet* 1989; 1: 721-2.
21. Sinha A, Nightingale J, West KP, *et al.* Epidermal growth factor enemas with oral mesalamine for mild-to-moderate left-sided ulcerative colitis or proctitis. *N Engl J Med* 2003; 349: 350-7.
22. Gionchetti P, Rizzello F, Morselli C, *et al.* Review article: problematic proctitis and distal colitis. *Aliment Pharmacol Ther* 2004; 20 Suppl 4: 93-6.
23. Lawrance IC, Copeland TS. Rectal tacrolimus in the treatment of resistant ulcerative proctitis. *Aliment Pharmacol Ther* 2008; 28: 1214-20.
24. van Dieren JM, van Bodegraven AA, Kuipers EJ, *et al.* Local application of tacrolimus in distal colitis: feasible and safe. *Inflamm Bowel Dis* 2009; 15: 193-8.
25. Bolin TD, Wong S, Crouch R, *et al.* Appendicectomy as a therapy for ulcerative proctitis. *Am J Gastroenterol* 2009; 104: 2476-82.
26. Bageacu S, Coatmeur O, Lemaitre JP, *et al.* Appendicectomy as a potential therapy for refractory ulcerative proctitis. *Aliment Pharmacol Ther* 2011; 34: 257-8.

Chapter 2

Management of left-sided ulcerative colitis

Joannie Ruel MD Assistant Professor of Medicine, Université de Sherbrooke, Faculty of Medicine, Division of Gastroenterology, Centre Hospitalier Universitaire de Sherbrooke, Québec, Canada

Sophie Plamondon MD FRCPC Assistant Professor of Medicine, Université de Sherbrooke, Faculty of Medicine, Division of Gastroenterology, Centre Hospitalier Universitaire de Sherbrooke, Québec, Canada; Centre de Recherche Étienne-LeBel, Québec, Canada

Overview

Left-sided or distal ulcerative colitis (UC) is defined as disease that extends no further than the splenic flexure. Approximately two thirds of patients with UC present with distal disease. The management of distal UC has been improved by the availability of a wide range of topical and oral 5-ASA agents, new drug formulations, multiple drug combinations and advances in immunosuppressive therapies. The recognition of symptom severity and extent of mucosal disease, and knowledge on the importance of mucosal healing and colorectal cancer prevention is essential for appropriate selection of therapy. The purpose of this chapter is to provide clinicians with an optimal management plan for the induction and maintenance of disease remission and an improvement in the quality of life, while reducing the need for long-term corticosteroids or surgery, and minimising colorectal cancer risk.

Introduction

Ulcerative proctosigmoiditis refers to disease involving the rectum and sigmoid colon. Left-sided or distal ulcerative colitis is defined as disease that extends from the rectum to the splenic flexure.

Around two-thirds of patients with ulcerative colitis (UC) present with either proctosigmoiditis or left-sided UC [1]. The risk of progression to the splenic flexure is 20% at 5 years for proctitis. Progression from distal disease to proximal disease (i.e. beyond the splenic flexure) occurs in up to 10% of patients at 10 years [2]. Up to 12% and 23% of patients with proctosigmoiditis and left-sided colitis, respectively, require colectomy after 25 years [3]. Risk factors for progression include disease severity, disease extent and younger age at diagnosis, presence of extra-intestinal manifestations (EIM), non-smoking status, ≥3 relapses per year and the need for systemic steroids or immunomodulators [3]. These data emphasize the need for prompt re-evaluation of disease extent if symptoms clinically worsen, even in patients with limited disease.

Clinical manifestations

Patients typically present with gradual onset of bloody diarrhoea, tenesmus and rectal urgency. Varying degrees of abdominal pain are often present. Presentation can be classified as mild, moderate or severe, based on the original Truelove-Witts criteria [4]. Most recent clinical trials have relied on other composite scores based on the number of daily soft stools, frequency of rectal bleeding, endoscopic appearance and physician global assessment (Mayo Clinic Index, Sutherland Index, UC Disease Activity Index) [5]. Severity correlates with the extent of disease. Fulminant disease is present at diagnosis in less than 10% of patients and is more common in extensive colitis or pancolitis. The diagnosis of UC is suspected on clinical grounds and supported by the appropriate findings on colonoscopy, histopathology and by negative stool examination for infectious causes.

Management (Figure 1)

Mild and moderate disease

Endoscopic extent and clinical severity determine the optimal approach to therapy. Therapeutic goals include rapid induction and maintenance of clinical remission, reduction in the need for long-term corticosteroids and decrease in colectomy and colorectal cancer incidence. Optimising quality of life is important. Functional impairment at school or work, and social and emotional support should also be assessed. Mucosal healing has emerged as an outcome measure in clinical trials of UC. Mucosal healing early in the disease course is associated with a significant reduction in the need for colectomy [6]. Endoscopic response at week eight predicts the likelihood of long-term remission on infliximab [7]. Patients with macroscopically normal mucosa may be less prone to dysplasia or

Left-sided UC
Confirm disease extent and activity with colonoscopy and histology

↓

Induction of remission

Mild/ moderate:	Combined oral and topical 5-ASA or steroids (enema)
Severe:	Oral/IV steroids and rescue therapies if steroid-refractory (refer to acute severe UC algorithm – Chapter 4)

↓

Maintenance of remission
Oral 5-ASA (+/- topical 5-ASA)
Oral 5-ASA and thiopurine if frequent relapser or steroid-refractory
Consider oral or topical tacrolimus, oral/IM methotrexate or anti-TNF drugs if thiopurine-refractory or intolerant

Figure 1. Proposed algorithm for left-sided ulcerative colitis.

colorectal cancer [8, 9]. The impact of mucosal healing on the natural history of the disease is still under investigation. Until further data become available, it is probably impractical to routinely assess for endoscopic remission. However, endoscopy is useful in patients who have not responded to therapy, or in those who wish to discontinue treatment.

5-aminosalicylic acid

5-aminosalicylic acid (5-ASA) drugs are the mainstay of therapy for mild to moderate distal UC. The exact mechanism of action of these compounds is uncertain, but may relate to enhanced peroxisome-proliferator activated receptor γ (PPAR-γ) gene expression, inhibition of prostaglandin and leucotriene synthesis, as well as IL-1 synthesis and NF-κB activation. 5-ASAs act topically and multiple formulations are now available to ensure proper colonic delivery and avoid proximal absorption of oral compounds through the small bowel.

Topical 5-ASA

The standard first-line induction therapy for distal UC involves topical 5-ASA drugs. They are superior to topical steroids or oral 5-ASA drugs alone in achieving clinical improvement [9, 10]. Topical 5-ASA drugs also have a more rapid effect than oral therapy. 5-ASA suppositories (500mg twice daily or 1000mg once daily) are effective as induction and maintenance treatment for proctitis [11, 12], whereas 5-ASA enemas (1 to 4g daily) reach the splenic flexure and are effective in inducing and maintaining remission in distal colitis [13, 14]. Remission rates are 78%, 72% and 65% when 5-ASA enemas are administered daily, every other day, or every third day, respectively [9].

Oral 5-ASA

Although topical therapy is highly effective for disease limited to the left colon, many patients find it inconvenient, and sometimes difficult to use.

Oral 5-ASAs are effective in inducing and maintaining remission in distal disease [15, 16]. In the past, sulfasalazine was used as first-line therapy. Sulfasalazine consists of a sulfapyridine moiety linked to a 5-ASA molecule through an azo-bond, which is cleaved by bacterial azoreductases upon reaching the colon. A similar strategy has been used with olsalazine and

Table 1. **Different oral and topical 5-ASA formulations.**

Agent	Formulation	Delivery	Dosing
Oral agents			
Sulfasalazine (500mg)	Sulfapyridine carrier	Colon	3-6g per day
Olsalazine (250mg)	5-ASA dimer	Colon	1.5-3g per day
Balsalazide (750mg)	Aminobenzoyl-alanine carrier	Colon	6.75g per day
Asacol (400, 800mg) Delayed release	Eudradigit S (pH 7)	Distal ileum, colon	2.4-4.8g per day
Salofalk (250, 500mg, 3g granule sachets) Delayed release	Eudradigit L (pH 6)	Ileum, colon	1.5-3g per day
Lialda (1.2g) Delayed release	Multimatrix (MMX)	Colon	2.4-4.8g per day
Pentasa (250, 500, 1000 2000mg) Sustained release	Ethylcellulose granules	Stomach, colon	2-4g per day
Topical agents			
Mesalamine suppository (400, 500, 1000mg)		Rectum	1-1.5g per day
Mesalamine enema (1.4g)	Suspension (50, 100ml)	Rectum Splenic flexure	1-4g per day to every 3 days

balsalazide, but these molecules contain benzoic acid instead of sulfapyridine, resulting in a more favourable side-effect profile.

Different 5-ASA formulations are shown in Table 1. The specific coat is dissolved through a pH-dependent or a delayed-release mechanism, allowing release of the active component in specific parts of the bowel. Traditionally, most preparations require multiple daily dosing, and the patient compliance rate is approximately 40%, which has a negative impact on both clinical and economic outcomes [17]. Recent studies have shown that once-daily high-dose administration of these compounds is as effective as the classical multiple-daily dosing options, for mesalamine 800mg (Asacol, Procter and Gamble Pharmaceuticals Ltd, Cincinnati, OH, USA), 1.2g (MMX mesalamine, Lialda, Shire, US), 2g (Pentasa, Ferring Pharmaceuticals Ltd, Wayne, PA, USA) and 3g granule sachets (Salofalk, Dr Falk Pharma UK Ltd, Bourne End, Buckinghamshire, UK; Freiburg, Germany).

Response to oral treatment is seen in 40-80% of patients within 2-4 weeks [9, 15]. As there are few comparative studies of different 5-ASAs, it is difficult to draw conclusions regarding their relative efficacy. Comparisons between studies are complicated by differences in definition of remission, study designs and endpoints. It is generally considered that the various formulations are equally effective. The combination of oral and topical 5-ASA is more effective than either alone [18]. This approach should be considered in patients with moderate disease.

A dose-response relationship has not been demonstrated consistently with all oral 5-ASA formulations, either as an induction or maintenance therapy. Recent large clinical trials have shown a dose response in patients with moderately active disease [19, 20]. However, for mild colitis, no advantage was seen for the higher dosing regimen in the 2.4-4.8g daily range. A higher induction dosage may be useful for a subgroup of difficult-to-treat moderate UC, especially those who have previously used two or more UC medications, including steroids, topical therapy or oral 5-ASAs [21].

Safety and tolerability

Intolerance to the sulfapyridine moiety of sulfasalazine is common, including nausea, vomiting, dyspepsia, anorexia and headache. Other adverse effects are abnormal sperm counts, drug-induced connective tissue disease and bone marrow suppression. Mesalamine is usually well tolerated. Side effects include allergic reactions, diarrhoea, pancreatitis, hepatotoxicity and interstitial nephritis. Serum creatinine should be monitored before initiating treatment and at 3-6 month intervals during the first year and then annually. Varying degrees of reversible thiopurine methyltransferase (TPMT) inhibition by 5-ASA drugs may be relevant in patients who are also receiving thiopurine therapy, leading to a theoretical risk of bone marrow suppression. However, the clinical effect of this interaction is probably modest.

Steroids

Topical steroids

Topical steroids (hydrocortisone 100mg or 10% hydrocortisone foam) may be used as induction therapy for distal colitis but not in the maintenance of remission, due to loss of efficacy over time and side effects generated by systemic absorption through the rectal mucosa. Budesonide enemas (2mg) which have a high hepatic first-pass metabolism seem to be as effective as the hydrocortisone preparation with less side effects [22].

Oral steroids

A recently developed formulation of MMX-budesonide designed for targeted colonic delivery has been shown to be effective in inducing remission of mild to moderate ulcerative colitis with minimal side effects (DDW 2011, A292, A746).

In patients with moderate to severe distal colitis refractory to maximal doses of 5-ASA drugs or, in those requiring rapid induction, oral steroids can be used. The recommended daily dose is 40-60mg of prednisone or an equivalent until clinical improvement and then weaned to zero over approximately 2 months.

Safety and tolerability

Adverse effects of corticosteroids include Cushingoid features, emotional and psychiatric disturbances, infections, glaucoma and cataracts, gastroduodenal mucosal injury, skin striae and impaired wound healing. Metabolic disturbances induced by corticosteroids are hyperglycaemia, sodium and fluid retention, hypokalaemia, metabolic alkalosis, hyperlipidaemia, accelerated atherogenesis and a risk of adrenal insufficiency. Osteopenia and osteoporosis are of particular concern.

Calcium supplementation and vitamin D should be added to corticosteroid therapy. Bisphosphonate therapy should be considered for long-term (>3 months) and recurrent steroid use, and for patients with a T-score below -2.5 on dual-energy X-ray absorptiometry or with other risk factors for osteoporosis.

Immunomodulators

In randomised controlled trials (RCTs) and uncontrolled series, thiopurines have been shown to be effective for steroid-dependent patients and can successfully prevent relapse in patients refractory to 5-ASA therapy [23, 24]. The recommended doses are 2-2.5mg/kg/d for azathioprine and 1-1.5mg/kg/d for 6-mercaptopurine (6-MP). As a result of their slow onset of action (3-6 months), these compounds are best used for maintenance of remission. They have steroid-sparing effects, and reduce both hospital admissions and colectomy rates [25].

Toxicities associated with thiopurines include bone marrow suppression, risk of opportunistic infections, liver abnormalities (2-17% of patients), allergic reactions (2-5%), pancreatitis (2%) and gastrointestinal intolerance. Thiopurines have been associated with a four-fold increase in the risk of lymphoma among IBD patients [26].

Thiopurines are metabolised to some of their inactive metabolites by thiopurine methyltransferase (TPMT). Around 0.3% of the general population has low to absent TPMT activity, leading to an increased production of the active metabolite, 6-TGN. Around 11% of patients have intermediate activity. TPMT genotyping or phenotyping is recommended before initiating thiopurine therapy to identify these patients, who are at high risk of early myelosuppression.

Measurement of metabolites such as 6-TGN and 6-MMP may help identify sub-therapeutic dosage, non-compliance and preferential metabolism to 6-MMP, which all contribute to clinical non-response. Further controlled trials are required for widespread use of these strategies.

Methotrexate

Controlled trials have failed to demonstrate efficacy of methotrexate in maintaining remission in UC. Methotrexate has therefore never been included in practice guidelines for UC. Some experts recommend its use in patients failing all other medical options and declining colectomy.

Anti-tumour necrosis factor-alpha therapy

Infliximab is reserved for patients who are steroid-refractory or steroid-dependent despite adequate doses of thiopurines or who are intolerant of these medications. It is also an option for severely active UC not responding to intravenous steroids.

Infliximab (5mg/kg) has been shown to be effective in inducing and maintaining remission in patients with moderate to severe UC failing corticosteroids and/or thiopurines (ACT 1) or 5-ASAs alone (ACT 2) [7]. Half to two-thirds of patients had left-sided ulcerative colitis. In ACT 1, 38.8% of patients were in remission at week 8, with 69.4% responding to therapy. Similar results were seen in ACT 2. Response and remission at week 54 were 45% and 42% in week-8 responders, when using a maintenance schedule of 5mg per kg intravenous infusion every 8 weeks. Steroid-free remission at week 54 was seen in 21% in the intention-to-treat population. Infliximab reduced the colectomy rate and the need for hospitalisation in moderately active UC at 54 weeks [27].

No prospective study has formally addressed whether concomitant thiopurine therapy would influence clinical response rates in UC. Clinical decision making should be individualised, taking into account the possibility of rare hepatosplenic T-cell lymphoma, especially in young males, with combination therapy.

Adverse effects of infliximab include infusion reactions, autoimmunity and increased risks of infection, lymphoma and possibly other malignancies, hepatotoxicity, development or exacerbation of multiple sclerosis or optic neuritis and worsening of congestive pre-existing heart failure. Infliximab is contraindicated in patients with these conditions, as well as active infection, untreated latent TB and current or recent malignancies.

Severe colitis

Few patients with distal colitis ultimately evolve to a severe refractory colitis. Treatment in such cases includes intravenous steroids. If no improvement is seen within 3-5 days, colectomy or treatment with intravenous cyclosporine or infliximab is recommended. A recent study published in abstract form has shown that cyclosporine and infliximab are equally effective, but infliximab is associated with a better side-effect profile (DDW 2011, A619) (see Chapter 4 for more details).

Surgery

Indications for surgery for distal UC are similar to more extensive forms. They include perforation, significant haemorrhage, dysplasia or carcinoma, severe colitis with or without megacolon unresponsive to conventional medical therapy and less severe but intractable symptoms or intolerable medication side effects. Total proctocolectomy with permanent ileostomy or ileal pouch-anal anastomosis (IPAA) are the two usual options (see Chapter 5 for more details).

Colorectal cancer (CRC) surveillance

Mucosal extent and duration of the inflammatory process determine the long-term risk of dysplasia and CRC, and guide the recommendations for endoscopic surveillance. The degree of risk is also associated with the degree of microscopic inflammation over time [28]. Patients with proctitis do not appear to be at increased risk. Left-sided UC is associated with a 2.8-fold increase in CRC risk compared with controls. Patients with primary sclerosing cholangitis (PSC) complicating UC have an increased risk of CRC. A family history must also be taken into account, as it increases the risk 2 to 4-fold [29].

Surveillance colonoscopy should be performed after 8-10 years of diagnosis according to American Gastroenterology Association (AGA) and British Society of Gastroenterology (BSG) guidelines, respectively, or as soon as a coexisting primary sclerosing cholangitis is identified. The optimal surveillance interval varies from 1-5 years in different guidelines, taking into account duration and extent of disease, as well as additional risk factors (family history, PSC, etc). The traditional approach of random biopsies (four biopsies every 10cm) is time-consuming and associated with a low pick-up rate. Current guidelines recommend surveillance with pancolonic dye spray and targeted biopsies [30, 31]. New techniques such as chromoendoscopy, magnification endoscopy and narrow-band imaging allow targeted screening biopsies. These advances are currently being investigated (see Chapter 16 for more details).

A meta-analysis and cohort studies suggested a chemopreventive effect of regular use of mesalamine with a 50% risk reduction of CRC and dysplasia [32]. The CESAME cohort also demonstrated the efficacy of thiopurine immunomodulators in reducing long-term colorectal cancer risk in IBD. The mechanism underlying these effects is thought to involve control of mucosal disease activity.

Conclusions

Left-sided ulcerative colitis is usually mild to moderate in intensity, but some patients may become refractory to standard therapy or progress to more proximal disease. The mainstay of therapy remains topical and oral 5-ASA drugs. Multiple new formulations have been developed in recent years to improve patient convenience and compliance. Immunomodulators may be necessary for moderate to severe, steroid-dependent or refractory disease. Infliximab has also been shown to be effective for induction and maintenance of remission in left-sided, refractory UC. Since it may reduce colorectal cancer risk and colectomy rates, early mucosal healing will likely become an important measure of response in clinical trials, and eventually a clinical treatment goal. Clinicians must remain aware of these new options and objectives to ensure optimal management of UC patients.

Key points

- **Two-thirds of UC patients present with distal disease.**
- **New formulations of 5-ASAs are available.**
- **Thiopurines are used for maintenance of remission in steroid-dependent and 5-ASA-refractory patients.**
- **Infliximab is effective in inducing and maintaining remission in patients with moderate to severe UC failing steroids, thiopurines or 5-ASAs alone.**
- **Early mucosal healing will become an important measure of response in clinical trials and eventually a clinical treatment goal.**

References

1. Farmer RG, Easly KA, Rankin GB. Clinical patterns, natural history, and progression of ulcerative colitis: a long-term follow-up of 1,116 patients. *Dig Dis Sci* 1993; 38: 1137-46.
2. Meucci G, Vecchi M, Astegiano M, *et al.* The natural history of ulcerative proctitis: a multicenter, retrospective study. *Am J Gastroenterol* 2000; 95: 469-73.
3. Langholz E, Munkholm P, Davidsen M, *et al.* Changes in the extent of ulcerative colitis - a study on the course and prognostic factors. *Scand J Gastroenterol* 1996; 31: 260.
4. Truelove SC, Witts LJ. Cortisone in ulcerative colitis; final report on a therapeutic trial. *Br Med J* 1955; 2: 1041-8.
5. D'Haens G, Sandborn WJ, Feagan BG, *et al.* A review of activity indices and efficacy end points for clinical trials of medical therapy in adults with ulcerative colitis. *Gastroenterology* 2007; 132: 763-86.
6. Froslie KF, Jahnsen J, Moum BA, *et al.* Mucosal healing in inflammatory bowel disease: results from a Norwegian population-based cohort. *Gastroenterology* 2007; 133: 412-22.
7. Rutgeerts P, Sandborn WJ, Feagan BG, *et al.* Infliximab for induction and maintenance therapy for ulcerative colitis. *N Engl J Med* 2005; 353(23): 2462-76.
8. Rutter M, Saunders B, Wilkinson K, *et al.* Severity of inflammation is a risk factor for colorectal neoplasia in ulcerative colitis. *Gastroenterology* 2004; 126: 451-9.
9. Cohen RD, Woseth DM, Thisted RA, *et al.* A meta-analysis and overview of the literature on treatment options for left-sided ulcerative colitis and ulcerative proctitis. *Am J Gastroenterol* 2000; 95: 1263-76.
10. Marshall JK, Irvine EJ. Rectal corticosteroids vs. alternative treatments in ulcerative colitis: a meta-analysis. *Gut* 1997; 40: 775-81.

11. Campieri M, De Franchis R, Bianchi Porro G, *et al.* Mesalazine (5-aminosalicylic acid) suppositories in the treatment of ulcerative proctitis or distal proctosigmoiditis. A randomized controlled trial. *Scand J Gastroenterol* 1990; 25: 663-8.
12. D'Arienzo A, Panarese A, D'Armiento FP, *et al.* 5-aminosalicylic acid suppositories in the maintenance of remission in idiopathic proctitis or proctosigmoiditis: a double-blind placebo-controlled clinical trial. *Am J Gastroenterol* 1990; 85: 1079-82.
13. Hanauer SB. Dose-ranging study of mesalamine (PENTASA) enemas in the treatment of acute ulcerative proctosigmoiditis: results of a multicentered placebo-controlled trial. The US PENTASA Enema Study Group. *Inflamm Bowel Dis* 1998; 4: 79-83.
14. Biddle WL, Greenberger NJ, Swan JT, *et al.* 5-aminosalicylic acid enemas: effective agent in maintaining remission in left-sided ulcerative colitis. *Gastroenterology* 1988; 94: 1075-9.
15. Sutherland L, Macdonald JK. Oral 5-aminosalicylic acid for induction of remission in ulcerative colitis. *Cochrane Database Syst Rev* 2006: CD000543.
16. Sutherland L, Macdonald JK. Oral 5-aminosalicylic acid for maintenance of remission in ulcerative colitis. *Cochrane Database Syst Rev* 2006: CD000544.
17. Kane, S, Huo D, Aikens J, *et al.* Medication non-adherence and the outcomes of patients with quiescent ulcerative colitis. *Am J Med* 2003; 114: 39-43.
18. Safdi M, DeMicco M, Sninsky C, *et al.* A double-blind comparison of oral vs. rectal mesalamine vs. combination therapy in the treatment of distal ulcerative colitis. *Am J Gastroenterol* 1997; 92: 1867-71.
19. Kamm MA, Lichtenstein GR, Sandborn WJ, *et al.* Randomised trial of once or twice-daily MMX mesalamine for maintenance of remission in ulcerative colitis. *Gut* 2008; 57: 893-902.
20. Hanauer SB, Sandborn WJ, Gassull M, *et al.* Delayed-release oral mesalamine at 4.8g/day for the treatment of moderately active ulcerative colitis: the ASCEND II trial. *Am J Gastroenterol* 2005; 100: 2478-85.
21. Lichstenstein GR, Kamm MA, Sandborn WJ, *et al.* MMX mesalazine for the induction of remission of mild-to-moderately active ulcerative colitis: efficacy and tolerability in specific patient subpopulations. *AP&T* 2008; 27(11): 1094-102.
22. Hanauer SB, Robinson M, Pruitt R, *et al.* Budesonide enema for the treatment of active, distal ulcerative colitis and proctitis: a dose-ranging study. US Budesonide Enema Study Group. *Gastroenterology* 1998; 115: 525-32.
23. Adler DJ, Korelitz BI. The therapeutic efficacy of 6-mercaptopurine in refractory ulcerative colitis. *Am J Gastroenterol* 1990; 85: 717-22.
24. Ardizzone S, Maconi G, Russo A, *et al.* Randomised controlled trial of azathioprine and 5-aminosalicylic acid for treatment of steroid-dependent ulcerative colitis. *Gut* 2006; 55: 47-53.
25. Gisbert JP, Nino P, Cara C, *et al.* Comparative effectiveness of azathioprine in Crohn's disease and ulcerative colitis: prospective, long-term, follow-up study of 394 patients. *Aliment Pharmacol Ther* 2008; 28: 228-38.
26. Beaugerie L, Brousse N, Bouvier AM, *et al*; CESAME Study Group. Lymphoproliferative disorders in patients receiving thiopurines for inflammatory bowel disease: a prospective observational cohort study. *Lancet* 2009; 374(9701): 1617-25.

27. Sandborn WJ, Rutgeerts P, Feagan BG, *et al.* Colectomy rate comparison after treatment of ulcerative colitis with placebo or infliximab. *Gastroenterology* 2009; 137: 1250-60.
28. Gupta RB, Harpaz N, Itzkowitz S, *et al.* Histologic inflammation is a risk factor for progression to colorectal neoplasia in ulcerative colitis: a cohort study. *Gastroenterol* 2007; 133: 1099-105.
29. Velayos FS, Loftus EV Jr, Jess T, *et al.* Predictive and protective factors associated with colorectal cancer in ulcerative colitis: a case-control study. *Gastroenterology* 2006; 130: 1941-9.
30. Cairns SR, Scholefield JH, Steele RJ, *et al.* Guidelines for colorectal carcinoma screening and surveillance in moderate to high risk groups (update from 2002). *Gut* 2010; 59: 666-89.
31. Farraye FA, Odze RD, Eaden J, *et al.* AGA medical position statement on the diagnosis and management of colorectal neoplasia in inflammatory bowel disease. *Gastroenterology* 2010; 138: 738-45.
32. Velayos FS, Terdiman JP, Walsh JM. Effect of 5-aminosalicylate use on colorectal cancer and dysplasia risk: a systematic review and meta-analysis of observational studies. *Am J Gastroenterol* 2005; 100: 1345-53.

Chapter 3

Management of extensive ulcerative colitis

Gwo-Tzer Ho MRCP PhD Consultant Gastroenterologist and MRC Clinician Scientist, University of Edinburgh, Western General Hospital, Edinburgh, Scotland

Craig Mowat MD FRCP Consultant Gastroenterologist, Ninewells Hospital and Medical School, Dundee, Scotland

Overview

Disease extent in ulcerative colitis (UC) determines the prognosis, risk of cancer and choice of therapy. Extensive UC is defined by involvement beyond the splenic flexure. Extensive UC has a distinct pathogenesis, clinical behaviour and disease progression. Patients with extensive UC have a higher risk of severe flare-up, corticosteroid resistance, more frequent need for admission to hospital, colectomy and colorectal cancer. This chapter reviews the clinical management of patients with extensive UC, which differs in some respects to patients with left-sided UC or proctitis.

Introduction

Extensive ulcerative colitis (UC) is generally defined according to the maximal macroscopic evidence of inflammation beyond the splenic flexure. The clinical presentation can be useful in evaluating disease extent in UC. In patients with disease limited to the rectosigmoid region, symptoms of rectal irritation, namely tenesmus (the sensation of incomplete emptying), small-volume diarrhoea and proximal constipation tend to predominate. In contrast, the clinical features of profuse bloody diarrhoea, abdominal cramping and systemic features such as general malaise, weight loss, fever and tachycardia are more prominent in patients with extensive or total UC.

At diagnosis, about 15% of patients have extensive colitis whilst 30% and 55% have left-sided colitis and proctitis, respectively. In a Danish population-based UC cohort (2003-2004), the prevalence of extensive UC at diagnosis was as high as 27% [1].

Extensive UC is associated with a stronger genetic contribution where the carriage of specific *HLA-DRB1* alleles and other common germline variants, for example, the *ABCB1/MDR1* gene, are higher. There is no gender predisposition and there are no known environmental factors that determine disease extent. Extensive UC is associated with more severe disease, an increased prevalence of corticosteroid resistance, the need for colectomy and colorectal malignancy. Primary sclerosing cholangitis (PSC) is associated with extensive UC although with milder disease severity. Therefore, clinical management of this entity requires further attention and differs in some respects to the management of UC as a whole.

Clinical progression of extensive UC

The management of UC is influenced by two key factors – disease extent and disease severity. These factors are closely linked, although not exclusively. In a UK series of 167 consecutive patients with acute severe UC (fulfilling Truelove and Witts criteria), 131 (81%) patients had extensive colonic involvement [2]. A review of selected hospital-based and population-based cohorts has shown that the risk of colectomy is strongly influenced by disease extent. The risk of colectomy among patients with only limited proctitis ranged from 2-9%, while patients with extensive colitis had 5-year colectomy rates of 30-44% [3-6]. More recent multicentre European data showed a three-fold increase in the risk of colectomy in patients with extensive disease, although with lower overall colectomy rates of 8.7% after 10-year follow-up [7]. A further inception cohort study showed that 50% of newly diagnosed patients with extensive UC who required corticosteroids at diagnosis, needed a colectomy at 1-year follow-up [8]. Finally, owing to the more aggressive clinical course of extensive UC, mortality is also higher in this group. In the Copenhagen County cohort (1967-1987), 23 (92%) of 25 patients who died due to UC-related complications, had extensive involvement [9]. Overall, patients with proctitis alone had a hazard ratio of 0.68 compared with those with extensive UC when adjusted for sex and age. A meta-analysis of ten population inception cohorts identified disease extent as the key factor for increased mortality in UC [10].

Disease extent, however, is not a static phenomenon. In a retrospective study of 145 patients with distal colitis at presentation, disease extension proximal to the sigmoid colon was 36% at a median of 6 years, becoming extensive in 29%. Using actuarial analysis, disease extension was predicted for 16% (95% CI, 11-24%) at 5 years and 31% (95% CI, 23-40%) 10 years after diagnosis [11]. In a further longitudinal population-based study, 30% of patients with limited disease progressed to more extensive disease after 5 years of follow-up [6], whereas in a cohort comprising 399 patients with UC, endoscopic regression occurred in 22% with histological regression in 24% [4]. Patients with extensive disease may have no clinical or histological evidence of colitis when in remission (indeed in this study, 30% of patients had a subsequently normal colonoscopy 14 months after diagnosis). These factors highlight the importance of re-evaluating disease extent and subsequent clinical management in the face of changing clinical patterns in UC.

Malignancy risk

Patients with UC have a higher risk of colorectal cancer (CRC) than the general population [12]. Disease extent and duration are the two critical factors underlying this association. Ekbom and colleagues reported standardised incidence ratios for CRC risk of 1.7 for patients with proctitis, 2.8 for patients with disease extending beyond the rectum but no further than the hepatic flexure, and 14.8 for patients with disease extending beyond the hepatic flexure [13]. The precise level of malignancy risk in this subset of patients is still under debate. In a large meta-analysis of 116 studies (1950-2000), Eaden and colleagues reported cumulative probabilities of CRC of 2% by 10 years, 8% by 20 years, and 18% by 30 years [12]. In a more recent study in the world's largest surveillance programme in patients with extensive UC to date (600 patients over a 30-year period), the cumulative incidence of CRC by disease duration was 2.5% at 20 years, 7.6% at 30 years and 10.8% at 40 years. In this study from St Mark's Hospital, London, only 30 of 600 patients (5%) developed CRC [14]. The reasons for such an improvement in the risk of CRC are not clear but may include improved control of mucosal inflammation, more extensive use of 5-ASA compounds, the implementation of surveillance programmes and timely colectomy.

Management (Figure 1)

Evaluation of disease extent

At diagnosis, objective evaluation of disease extent should be carried out as soon and safely as possible. The gold standard for assessment of disease extent is combined colonoscopy and histological examination. Colonoscopy is not generally recommended in acute severe colitis. In this setting, a simple non-invasive test such as a plain abdominal X-ray, that demonstrates an empty and/or oedematous colon in the affected regions, can be a useful guide to determine disease extent. Patients with severe disease regardless of disease extent (as defined by Truelove and Witts criteria: >6 bloody stools/day with one or more of these features: fever, resting tachycardia, anaemia or elevated inflammatory markers) will

Extensive UC
Confirm disease extent and activity with colonoscopy and histology

↓

Induction of remission

Mild:	Oral 5-ASA
Moderate:	Combined oral and topical 5-ASA and early introduction of steroids
Severe:	Oral/IV steroids and rescue therapies if steroid-refractory (refer to acute severe UC algorithm – Chapter 4)

↓

Maintenance of remission
Oral 5-ASA alone
Oral 5-ASA and thiopurine if frequent relapser or steroid-refractory
Consider tacrolimus, methotrexate, leucocytapheresis or anti-TNF drugs if thiopurine-refractory or intolerant
Surveillance colonoscopy according to guidelines (refer to surveillance algorithm – Chapter 16)

Figure 1. Proposed algorithm for extensive ulcerative colitis.

require hospital admission for joint medical/surgical management (see Chapter 4).

Complications and the need for colectomy usually occur within the first 2 years of diagnosis; these outcomes are directly linked to extensive disease. Clinical trials, however, do not stratify patients according to disease extent but rather, disease activity.

Induction of remission

The need for rapid control of active disease in patients with extensive UC is important. In general, the management for moderate to severe extensive UC is similar to that of left-sided disease, but there should be a lower threshold for treatment with steroids. Higher mesalazine doses can be used but close monitoring is essential as some patients may progress rapidly to acute severe disease. Poorly controlled disease is associated with an increased risk of complications, including toxic dilatation. At present, there are no consistent clinical or biological markers to predict patients that will progress to severe disease.

Mesalazine

5-aminosalicylic acids (ASA) or mesalazine preparations remain the cornerstone of medical treatment. The dose response is more important than the type of 5-ASA preparations used:

- Oral mesalazine 2.0-4.8g daily or balsalazide 6.75g (delivering 2.4g mesalazine) daily are effective first-line therapy for mild-moderately active extensive disease.
- The combination of oral and rectal (enema) formulations of mesalazine leads to faster and higher remission rates [15]. In addition, rectal preparations may help symptoms relating to rectal irritation.
- Once daily dosing with mesalazine is at least as effective as conventional dosing regimes [16].

Corticosteroids

- Prednisolone 40mg daily is appropriate for patients with moderately active disease, in whom mesalazine in appropriate dose and route has been unsuccessful. As the median time for 5-ASA response is 2-4 weeks, oral corticosteroids can be introduced at 4 weeks following 5-ASA treatment if no response is evident. However, in the face of rapid clinical deterioration, an earlier introduction may be warranted. Depending on clinical condition and patient choice, the use of higher-dose 5-ASA (e.g. ≥4g/day) is a further option before committing patients to corticosteroids. Prednisolone is also appropriate in patients who relapse despite a maintenance dose of 5-ASA. Prednisolone should be reduced gradually according to severity and patient response, generally over 8 weeks. There are no randomised trials comparing different tapering strategies. Most physicians reduce dosage by 5mg/week and our local experience suggests that more rapid reduction is associated with early relapse. The likelihood of early relapse, sub-optimal response or lack of response to corticosteroids is higher in patients with extensive and severe UC than those with distal disease.

- Budesonide (colonic release preparation) appears as effective as prednisolone for mild-moderate extensive colitis.

Rescue therapies (infliximab or cyclosporine)

In the acute severe UC setting, the use of second-line medical therapies, namely cyclosporine and infliximab can be used and are considered briefly here. Intravenous cyclosporine induces remission in 60-80% of patients with severe active UC [17]. The ACT-1/2 study demonstrated the efficacy of infliximab in active UC with superior response and remission rates at week 8 [18]. Jarnerot *et al* demonstrated that a single infusion of infliximab at 5mg/kg was effective rescue therapy in hospitalised patients with acute severe UC failing to respond to first-line intensive medical therapy ($p=0.017$, odds ratio 4.7)[19]. The current strategy and positioning of infliximab, as with cyclosporine, is to use this as a 'bridge' to longer-term immunosuppressive maintenance treatment such as azathioprine. The management of acute severe UC has been discussed in detail in Chapter 4.

Maintenance of remission

Mesalazine

The British Society of Gastroenterology and the European Crohn's and Colitis Organisation guidelines advocate the use of 5-ASA to maintain remission in all patients with UC, including those with extensive disease [20, 21]. Few studies have focused on disease extent *per se* as a risk factor for disease relapse. Nevertheless, in pragmatic terms, patients with extensive disease have more to benefit from maintenance 5-ASA treatment. Conversely, poorly controlled extensive disease will incur a greater risk of complications to the patient and a higher burden on health resources. Although, a Cochrane Review suggested that dosage of 5-ASA >1.2g/day conferred no additional benefit, a further study showed that a higher dose was more effective in preventing relapse in patients with extensive disease [21, 22]. Oral mesalazine 1.2g-2.4g daily or balsalazide 4.5g daily should be considered as first-line therapy to maintain remission. Longer-term topical 5-ASA therapy is effective; however, this option is not generally preferred by patients. Adherence to 5-ASA is essential in the maintenance of remission; simpler once-daily dosing regimens are more acceptable.

Immunosuppression

Azathioprine (AZA)/mercaptopurine (MP) is recommended for patients who have early or frequent relapses while taking an optimal dose of 5-ASA or in patients who are intolerant of 5-ASA. AZA/MP is effective in patients with steroid-dependent or refractory disease or in those with poor disease control and frequent relapses on 5-ASA alone [23]. In these patients, most physicians will use thiopurine drugs in combination with 5-ASA, given the potential protective effect of 5-ASA drugs on colorectal cancer.

Anti-TNF therapy

The benefit of infliximab in UC is unclear. Whilst the ACT1/2 achieved their primary endpoints, corticosteroid-free remission after a year of 8-weekly infliximab infusion was observed in only 21% of the patients. Colectomy rates at 54 weeks have recently been published and showed only an absolute risk reduction of 7% in the infliximab treated group (10% vs. 17% in infliximab and placebo, respectively) [24]. Approximately 45% of ACT1/2 patients have extensive disease; the hazard ratio for colectomy in patients for extensive UC was 1.23 (95% CI, 0.78-1.94) compared with left-sided UC.

In patients who are refractory to conventional management yet do not exhibit features of progressive severe disease, methotrexate, calcineurin inhibitors, leucocytapheresis or elective surgery for chronic continuous symptoms can be considered.

Longstanding disease and malignancy screening

Colonoscopic surveillance is indicated in patients with extensive UC. In the recently updated BSG guideline (see Chapter 16), all patients with UC should receive a colonoscopic evaluation at 10 years to determine disease extent and endoscopic risk factors [25]. The current gold standard includes pancolonic dye-spraying with targeted biopsies rather than random biopsies. Surveillance intervals at 5, 3 and 1-year have been defined by risks rather than disease duration (see Chapter 16).

Regular patient-physician review is essential to ensure compliance. A case-control study by Eaden *et al* showed a relative reduction of 75% and 84% in risk of cancer in patients taking regular 5-ASA and in those receiving bi-annual physician review, respectively [26]. Prompt treatment, swift attention to changing clinical symptoms and good patient education are relevant factors in the management of this group of patients.

Conclusions

Extensive UC has an aggressive clinical course and a high risk of complications. However, more recent studies based on outcomes such as colectomy, colorectal cancer and mortality have shown encouraging trends of improvement likely to be secondary to better understanding, health-care delivery and the general management of UC.

Key points

- Extensive UC affects the colon beyond the splenic flexure.
- 15-30% of patients with UC have extensive involvement.
- Extensive UC is associated with more severe disease, an increased prevalence of corticosteroid resistance, the need for colectomy and colorectal malignancy.
- Disease extent is not a static phenomenon and changes over time.
- The clinical management for active extensive UC is similar to that of left-sided disease but with a lower threshold for the introduction of corticosteroids.
- Combined oral and topical 5-ASA is more effective than the oral preparation alone.
- Thiopurines (azathioprine and 6-mercaptopurine) are effective maintenance therapy for patients with UC who have failed or cannot tolerate mesalazine and for patients who require repeated courses of steroids.
- In patients who fail or cannot tolerate thiopurines, other immunomodulators (calcineurin inhibitors, methotrexate), leucocytapheresis or anti-TNF drugs can be considered but a surgical opinion should also be sought.

References

1. Jess T, Riis L, Vind I, *et al.* Changes in clinical characteristics, course, and prognosis of inflammatory bowel disease during the last 5 decades: a population-based study from Copenhagen, Denmark. *Inflamm Bowel Dis* 2007; 13: 481-9.
2. Ho GT, Mowat C, Goddard CJ, *et al.* Predicting the outcome of severe ulcerative colitis: development of a novel risk score to aid early selection of patients for second-line medical therapy or surgery. *Aliment Pharmacol Ther* 2004; 19(10): 1079-87.
3. Ritchie JK, Powell-Tuck J, Lennard-Jones JE. Clinical outcome of the first ten years of ulcerative colitis and proctitis. *Lancet* 1978; 1(8074): 1140-3.

4. Moum B, Ekbom A, Vatn MH, *et al.* Clinical course during the 1st year after diagnosis in ulcerative colitis and Crohn's disease. Results of a large, prospective population-based study in southeastern Norway, 1990-93. *Scand J Gastroenterol* 1997; 32(10): 1005-12.
5. Farmer RG, Easley KA, Rankin GB. Clinical patterns, natural history, and progression of ulcerative colitis. A long-term follow-up of 1116 patients. *Dig Dis Sci* 1993; 38: 1137-46.
6. Langholz E, Munkholm P, Davidsen M, Binder V. Course of ulcerative colitis: analysis of changes in disease activity over years. *Gastroenterology* 1994; 107: 3-11.
7. Hoie O, Wolters FL, Riis L, *et al.* Low colectomy rates in ulcerative colitis in an unselected European cohort followed for 10 years. *Gastroenterology* 2007; 132: 507-15.
8. Ho GT, Chiam P, Drummond H, *et al.* The efficacy of corticosteroid therapy in inflammatory bowel disease: analysis of a 5-year UK inception cohort. *Aliment Pharmacol Ther* 2006; 24: 319-30.
9. Winther KV, Jess T, Langholz E, *et al.* Survival and cause-specific mortality in ulcerative colitis: follow-up of a population-based cohort in Copenhagen County. *Gastroenterology* 2003; 125: 1576-82.
10. Jess T, Gamborg M, Munkholm P, Sorensen TI. Overall and cause-specific mortality in ulcerative colitis: meta-analysis of population-based inception cohort studies. *Am J Gastroenterol* 2007; 102: 609-17.
11. Ayres RC, Gillen CD, Walmsley RS, Allan RN. Progression of ulcerative proctosigmoiditis: incidence and factors influencing progression. *Eur J Gastroenterol Hepatol* 1996; 8: 555-8.
12. Eaden JA, Abrams KR, Mayberry JF. The risk of colorectal cancer in ulcerative colitis: a meta-analysis. *Gut* 2001; 48: 526-35.
13. Ekbom A, Helmick C, Zack M, Adami HO. Ulcerative colitis and colorectal cancer. A population-based study. *N Engl J Med* 1990; 323(18): 1228-33.
14. Rutter MD, Saunders BP, Wilkinson KH, *et al.* Thirty-year analysis of a colonoscopic surveillance program for neoplasia in ulcerative colitis. *Gastroenterology* 2006; 130: 1030-8.
15. Marteau P, Probert CS, Lindgren S, *et al.* Combined oral and enema treatment with Pentasa (mesalazine) is superior to oral therapy alone in patients with extensive mild/moderate active ulcerative colitis: a randomised, double blind, placebo controlled study. *Gut* 2005; 54: 960-5.
16. Dignass AU, Bokemeyer B, Adamek H, *et al.* Mesalamine once daily is more effective than twice daily in patients with quiescent ulcerative colitis. *Clin Gastroenterol Hepatol* 2009; 7: 762-9.
17. Lichtiger S, Present DH, Kornbluth A, *et al.* Cyclosporine in severe ulcerative colitis refractory to steroid therapy. *N Engl J Med* 1994; 330(26): 1841-5.
18. Rutgeerts P, Sandborn WJ, Feagan BG, *et al.* Infliximab for induction and maintenance therapy for ulcerative colitis. *N Engl J Med* 2005; 353(23): 2462-76.
19. Jarnerot G, Hertervig E, Friis-Liby I, *et al.* Infliximab as rescue therapy in severe to moderately severe ulcerative colitis: a randomized, placebo-controlled study. *Gastroenterology* 2005; 128: 1805-11.

20. Mowat C, Cole A, Windsor A, *et al.* Guidelines for the management of inflammatory bowel disease in adults. *Gut* 2011; 60: 571-607.
21. Sutherland L, Macdonald JK. Oral 5-aminosalicylic acid for maintenance of remission in ulcerative colitis. *Cochrane Database Syst Rev* 2006; 2: CD000544.
22. Paoluzi OA, Iacopini F, Pica R, *et al.* Comparison of two different daily dosages (2.4 vs. 1.2g) of oral mesalazine in maintenance of remission in ulcerative colitis patients: 1-year follow-up study. *Aliment Pharmacol Ther* 2005; 21: 1111-9.
23. Ardizzone S, Maconi G, Russo A, *et al.* Randomised controlled trial of azathioprine and 5-aminosalicylic acid for treatment of steroid-dependent ulcerative colitis. *Gut* 2006; 55: 47-53.
24. Sandborn WJ, Rutgeerts P, Feagan BG, *et al.* Colectomy rate comparison after treatment of ulcerative colitis with placebo or infliximab. *Gastroenterology* 2009; 137: 1250-60.
25. Cairns SR, Scholefield JH, Steele RJ, *et al.* Guidelines for colorectal cancer screening and surveillance in moderate and high risk groups (update from 2002). *Gut* 2010; 59: 666-89.
26. Eaden J, Abrams K, Ekbom A, *et al.* Colorectal cancer prevention in ulcerative colitis: a case-control study. *Aliment Pharmacol Ther* 2000; 14: 145-53.

Chapter 4

Acute severe ulcerative colitis

Siew Ng MBBS PhD MRCP Assistant Professor, Institute of Digestive Disease, Department of Medicine and Therapeutics, Chinese University of Hong Kong, Hong Kong; Senior Lecturer and Honorary Gastroenterologist, St Vincent's Hospital, University of Melbourne, Australia

Ailsa L. Hart BMBCh MRCP PhD Senior Clinical Lecturer, Imperial College and Consultant Gastroenterologist, St Mark's Hospital, London, UK

Overview

Acute severe ulcerative colitis (UC) is associated with high mortality. Management requires a proactive and time-bound approach between physicians and surgeons. Intravenous corticosteroids remain the first-line therapy. In patients not responding after 3-5 days of steroids, the use of rescue therapy with low-dose intravenous cyclosporine or intravenous infliximab 5mg/kg should be considered. Controlled data suggest that cyclosporine and infliximab have comparable efficacy in the short term. In thiopurine-naïve patients, cyclosporine is effective as a bridge to the effect of azathioprine or 6-mercaptopurine. In those exposed to thiopurine, infliximab may be more favourable for its short-term safety profile and the option of long-term maintenance treatment. Cyclosporine and infliximab prevent colectomy in at least half of the patients in the long term. However, medical rescue therapy should not defer the indication for colectomy in those with an inadequate response.

Introduction

Acute severe ulcerative colitis (UC) affects 15% of patients with UC at some point in their disease course [1]. Hospitalisation should be considered in patients passing more than six bloody stools per day associated with fever, tachycardia, anaemia and raised C-reactive protein (CRP) or ESR [2]. Upon admission, enteric infection should be carefully excluded. Patients presenting with *Clostridium difficile* infection complicating acute severe UC have an increased risk of colectomy and mortality [3], and should be treated with antibiotics, such as metronidazole or vancomycin [4]. An unprepared flexible sigmoidoscopy with minimal air insufflation and mucosal biopsies by an experienced endoscopist are helpful to assess the severity of inflammation and to exclude cytomegalovirus (CMV) infection.

Table 1. Assessing and managing acute severe UC.

- Establish a case of severe acute UC based on Truelove and Witts criteria
- Stool cultures to exclude infectious causes of colitis including *Clostridium difficile*
- Abdominal radiography to exclude toxic megacolon
- Prophylactic subcutaneous heparin to reduce the risk of thromboembolism
- Intravenous fluid replacement with potassium supplementation
- Dietition review and calorie supplementation for malnourished patients
- Blood transfusions to maintain the Hb >10g/dL
- Avoid opioids, non-steroidal anti-inflammatory drugs and anti-cholinergic drugs

Even though the precise role of active CMV infection in acute severe UC is still debated, the presence of CMV inclusion bodies on biopsies should prompt treatment with ganciclovir, especially in patients slow to respond to conventional therapy. Daily monitoring and optimisation of the overall supportive care of patients with acute severe UC is crucial for improved outcomes (Table 1). Response to intravenous corticosteroids should be assessed between days 3 to 5. In cases of non-response with worsening stool frequency, CRP, serum albumin levels or abdominal radiography, rescue therapies with intravenous cyclosporine or intravenous infliximab should be considered. However, complications including toxic megacolon together with clinical deterioration require emergency colectomy. The decision of rescue therapy or surgery should involve a multidisciplinary approach between gastroenterologist, surgeon, dietician and stomatherapist.

Corticosteroids

In acute severe UC, the first-line therapy is corticosteroids [5, 6], and the overall response rate to steroids is 67% [7]. The introduction of steroids has reduced mortality from 50% to less than 10% [5, 8]. In patients not responding (>8 stools per day or 3-8 stools per day plus a CRP >45mg/L) after 3 days of corticosteroids, the colectomy rate rises to 85% [9]. In the short term, approximately one-third of patients fails to respond to steroids and require rescue medical therapies or surgery.

Cyclosporine

Cyclosporine, the fungal calcineurin inhibitor, has been shown to be an effective rescue therapy for acute severe UC in two controlled trials. In the study by Lichtiger *et al*, nine out of 11 patients responded to cyclosporine (4mg/kg for a mean of 7 days) and zero out of nine patients responded to placebo in the short term [10]. Van Assche *et al* showed in a single-centre controlled study that response rate at day 8 was comparable between cyclosporine 2mg/kg (86%) and 4mg/kg (84%) [11]. Cyclosporine is also effective in patients with severe acute UC before failure of corticosteroids [12]. Pooled results from controlled and

Part 1

uncontrolled trials showed that 76-85% of patients will respond to intravenous cyclosporine and avoid colectomy in the short term [10, 11, 13]. Following initial response to cyclosporine, about 50% will avoid colectomy at 3 years [14]. On longer-term follow-up, the probability of avoiding colectomy after successful intravenous cyclosporine therapy was 41% at 4 years, 16% at 6 years and 12% at 7 years [15]. Oral cyclosporine is also effective in the treatment of acute severe UC [16], but data are based on retrospective uncontrolled studies [17]. Once cyclosporine has been initiated, drug levels should be monitored on day 2-3 and dosage should be adjusted to the levels of 150-300ng/ml [16, 18]. Several predictors of poor response to cyclosporine have been reported (Figure 1) [19, 20, 11]. Azathioprine improves the long-term efficacy of cyclosporine [13]. In patients who had an initial response to cyclosporine, response increased to 71% in those who were treated with azathioprine or 6-mercaptopurine (6-MP), compared with 55% in those who were on cyclosporine alone.

Infliximab

Jarnerot *et al* investigated the efficacy of infliximab as rescue therapy in 45 patients with moderately severe UC not responding to intravenous corticosteroids. Significantly more patients who had placebo (67%) required colectomy than those who had a single dose of infliximab (29%) [21]. The greatest benefit to infliximab was seen in patients who had severe or moderately severe but not fulminant UC. Several uncontrolled studies have shown that infliximab prevents colectomy in approximately three-quarters of patients at 1 year [22, 23], and in 50% of the patients at 2-3 years [24-26]. Overall, infliximab is effective in preventing colectomy in acute severe UC in the short term and the response may be durable. Figure 1 shows the predictors of colectomy with infliximab [27, 28].

Choosing between cyclosporine or infliximab

In a recent multicentre randomised controlled trial, the GETAID group compared the efficacy of infliximab versus cyclosporine in patients with

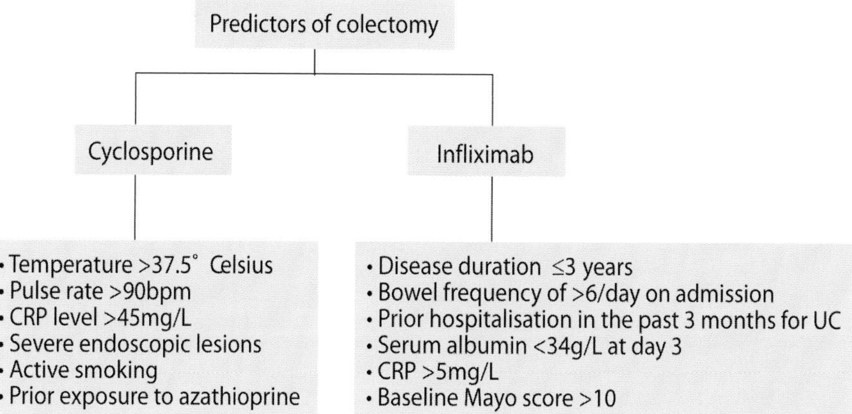

Figure 1. Predictors of colectomy in patients with acute severe UC treated with cyclosporine and infliximab.

acute severe UC refractory to intravenous steroids. The primary endpoint was the rate of treatment failure defined by: absence of clinical response at day 7; absence of remission (Mayo score ≤2 without any subscore >1) without steroids at day 98; relapse between day 7 and day 98; severe adverse event leading to treatment interruption; colectomy and fatality. One hundred and eleven patients with acute severe UC (Lichtiger score ≥10) refractory to intravenous steroids were randomised to either intravenous cyclosporine (2mg/kg/d for 1 week, then switched orally during 98 days), or infliximab (5mg/kg at weeks 0, 2 and 6). In patients with clinical response at day 7, azathioprine was

Table 2. Medical rescue therapies for acute severe UC.

	Cyclosporine	Infliximab
Dosing	• 2 (to 4)mg/kg intravenous • 5mg/kg oral • Aim serum trough level 150-300	• IV 5mg/kg week 0, 2 and 6, and every 8 weeks
Onset of action	• Median 4 days	• After one dose
Efficacy	• Short term 76-85% • 3 years 50% colectomy-free • 7 years 12% colectomy-free	• Short term 66-85% • 3 years 50% colectomy-free
Complications	• Seizure • Anaphylaxis • Serious infections • Nephrotoxicity • Neurotoxicity	• Serious infections • Anaphylaxis
Ways to limit side effects	• Use 2mg instead of 4mg [11, 18] • Monitor magnesium and cholesterol levels • Consider oral formulation (especially if magnesium or cholesterol levels are low) • Rapid weaning of steroids • Minimise concomitant immunosuppressant use • Prophylaxis with cotrimoxazole in patients on triple immunomodulators	• Rapid weaning of steroids • Temporary diverting ileostomy in patients requiring surgery

started at a dose of 2.5mg/kg/d and steroids were decreased according to a fixed regimen. Treatment failure rates (60% versus 54%), response rates at day 7 (84% versus 86%), and mucosal healing rates (52% versus 53%) were comparable between cyclosporine and infliximab groups. At day 98, 10 patients treated with cyclosporine and 13 with infliximab had a colectomy. Ten severe adverse events were observed in nine patients with cyclosporine and 16 in 16 patients with infliximab. More patients on infliximab had disease worsening [29], but there were no deaths. The decision to use infliximab or cyclosporine depends on an assessment of the patient's previous exposure to immunomodulators, the side-effect profiles of the drug and combined physician and patient choice. Cyclosporine with a bridge to azathioprine is most effective in patients naïve to thiopurine. In contrast, in patients presenting with a severe episode of UC whilst maintained on optimal-dose azathioprine, infliximab is probably more useful as induction and maintenance therapy [15]. However, consideration for early surgery may be more appropriate. In patients who were already on immunomodulators at the time of admission with acute severe UC, the likelihood of needing a colectomy following treatment with cyclosporine is high. Table 2 summarises the use of cyclosporine and infliximab as rescue therapies.

Switching between cyclosporine and infliximab

Several uncontrolled studies have reported the consecutive use of cyclosporine and infliximab in patients with acute severe UC. A study from Mount Sinai New York of 19 patients with fulminant UC suggested that patients receiving infliximab followed by cyclosporine or vice versa have an increased risk of sepsis and mortality [30]. In the largest study by a French collaborative group of 86 patients, 62% of patients who received both drugs consecutively avoided colectomy in the short term but at 3 years colectomy rates were 63%. About one-third of patients had adverse effects consisting mostly of infections [31]. In a smaller Spanish study, 16 patients with acute UC were treated with infliximab after failing cyclosporine; 38% of patients required a colectomy in the short term [32]. Theoretically it is safer to use infliximab after cyclosporine than to use these drugs in the reverse order in view of the shorter half-life of cyclosporine. Nonetheless even if the half-life of cyclosporine is less than 24 hours, the impact on the risk of infection may still be long-lasting.

Adverse effects of cyclosporine and infliximab

Both cyclosporine and infliximab are associated with an increased risk of serious opportunistic infections [33]. Previous steroid exposure adds to the toxicity [34]. In a long-term study of the TREAT Registry with a follow-up of 4.8 years, infliximab-treated patients showed an increased risk of serious infections compared with non-infliximab treated patients [35]. A study from Edinburgh showed that major complications and mortality rate was 5.2% and 2.6%, respectively, in patients with acute UC treated with infliximab [28]. Switching between infliximab and cyclosporine is associated with serious adverse effects and death, and is not recommended as a standard approach [30, 31]. A risk/benefit analysis of medical therapy needs to be compared with 'curative' surgery which carries a mortality of about 3% in the early postoperative period. Both short-term and long-term post-colectomy mortality is substantially reduced when an elective, and not an emergency colectomy, is performed.

Surgery

Early post-colectomy mortalities have been reported to be around 2-3% of patients with acute severe UC [36, 37]. Colectomy should not be delayed for more than 5 days in patients with inadequate response as delayed colectomy is associated with increased in-hospital mortality [38]. Short-term mortality after surgery for UC was lower in those who underwent elective surgery than those who had emergency surgery [38-42]. Age greater than 50 years old at admission, male gender, comorbidity, hospital stay beyond 2 weeks, and prior hospital admission for IBD were independently associated with mortality [42]. Furthermore, patients who had a significantly longer duration of pre-operative medical therapy were more likely to have major postoperative complications [43].

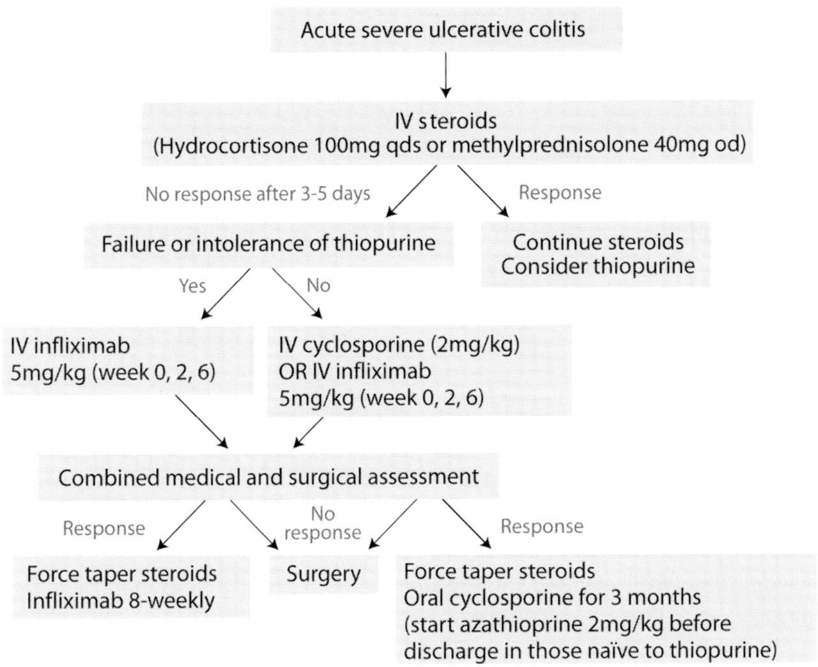

Figure 2. Proposed algorithm for the treatment of patients with acute severe UC.

Delayed surgery for patients who do not respond to medical therapy is associated with an increased risk of postoperative complications [43]. A meta-analysis showed that pre-operative infliximab use increased the risk of total short-term postoperative complications (OR 1.8) which included wound infection, sepsis and abscess [44]. A total colectomy and ileostomy, with the rectum left *in situ* is recommended in those who need surgery. Reconstructive surgery is best performed approximately 6 months after primary surgery [45]. A detailed discussion of surgery in ulcerative colitis is in Chapter 5.

Conclusions

Intravenous steroids remain first-line therapy for acute severe UC. Patients who do not respond to corticosteroids within 3 days should be considered for rescue medical therapy with either intravenous cyclosporine or infliximab. The decision should be based on the patient's previous immunosuppressant history, age, and comorbidity. Surgery may be unavoidable in some patients and optimal management requires close collaboration between the gastroenterologist and the surgeon. Patients who are naïve to thiopurines should be started on thiopurine during the acute admission when treated with intravenous cyclosporine to optimise long-term outcome and avoid colectomy. If a patient presenting with acute severe UC is already taking a thiopurine at the time of admission, the outcome with cyclosporine is less favourable and infliximab or early surgery need to be considered.

A proposed algorithm for the treatment of acute severe UC is shown in Figure 2.

Key points

- **Fifteen percent of patients with UC will have a severe acute attack that requires admission to hospital.**
- **Cyclosporine and infliximab are effective as rescue therapies in intravenous steroid-refractory acute severe UC.**
- **Approximately 75% and 50% of patients treated with cyclosporine avoid colectomy in the short and long term, respectively.**
- **Serious opportunistic infections are associated with medical rescue therapies.**

References

1. Edwards FC, Truelove SC. The course and prognosis of ulcerative colitis. *Gut* 1963; 4: 299-315.
2. Truelove SC, Witts LJ. Cortisone in ulcerative colitis; preliminary report on a therapeutic trial. *Br Med J* 1954; 2: 375-8.
3. Jodorkovsky D, Young Y, Abreu MT. Clinical outcomes of patients with ulcerative colitis and co-existing *Clostridium difficile* infection. *Dig Dis Sci* 2010; 55: 415-20.
4. Ananthakrishnan AN, Issa M, Binion DG. *Clostridium difficile* and inflammatory bowel disease. *Med Clin North Am* 2010; 94: 135-53.
5. Truelove SC, Witts LJ. Cortisone in ulcerative colitis; final report on a therapeutic trial. *Br Med J* 1955; 2: 1041-8.
6. Truelove SC, Jewell DP. Intensive intravenous regimen for severe attacks of ulcerative colitis. *Lancet* 1974; 1: 1067-70.
7. Turner D, Walsh CM, Steinhart AH, *et al.* Response to corticosteroids in severe ulcerative colitis: a systematic review of the literature and a meta-regression. *Clin Gastroenterol Hepatol* 2007; 5: 103-10.
8. Jakobovits SL, Travis SP. Management of acute severe colitis. *Br Med Bull* 2005; 75-76: 131-44.
9. Travis SP, Farrant JM, Ricketts C, *et al.* Predicting outcome in severe ulcerative colitis. *Gut* 1996; 38: 905-10.
10. Lichtiger S, Present DH, Kornbluth A, *et al.* Cyclosporine in severe ulcerative colitis refractory to steroid therapy. *N Engl J Med* 1994; 330: 1841-5.
11. Van Assche G, D'Haens G, Noman M, *et al.* Randomized, double-blind comparison of 4mg/kg versus 2mg/kg intravenous cyclosporine in severe ulcerative colitis. *Gastroenterology* 2003; 125: 1025-31.
12. D'Haens G, Lemmens L, Geboes K, *et al.* Intravenous cyclosporine versus intravenous corticosteroids as single therapy for severe attacks of ulcerative colitis. *Gastroenterology* 2001; 120: 1323-9.
13. Cohen RD, Stein R, Hanauer SB. Intravenous cyclosporin in ulcerative colitis: a five-year experience. *Am J Gastroenterol* 1999; 94: 1587-92.
14. Arts J, D'Haens G, Zeegers M, *et al.* Long-term outcome of treatment with intravenous cyclosporin in patients with severe ulcerative colitis. *Inflamm Bowel Dis* 2004; 10: 73-8.
15. Moskovitz DN, Van AG, Maenhout B, *et al.* Incidence of colectomy during long-term follow-up after cyclosporine-induced remission of severe ulcerative colitis. *Clin Gastroenterol Hepatol* 2006; 4: 760-5.
16. Campbell S, Travis S, Jewell D. Ciclosporin use in acute ulcerative colitis: a long-term experience. *Eur J Gastroenterol Hepatol* 2005; 17: 79-84.
17. Fellermann K, Tanko Z, Herrlinger KR, *et al.* Response of refractory colitis to intravenous or oral tacrolimus (FK506). *Inflamm Bowel Dis* 2002; 8: 317-24.
18. Rayner CK, McCormack G, Emmanuel AV, *et al.* Long-term results of low-dose intravenous ciclosporin for acute severe ulcerative colitis. *Aliment Pharmacol Ther* 2003; 18: 303-8.

19. Cacheux W, Seksik P, Lemann M, *et al.* Predictive factors of response to cyclosporine in steroid-refractory ulcerative colitis. *Am J Gastroenterol* 2008; 103: 637-42.
20. Rowe FA, Walker JH, Karp LC, *et al.* Factors predictive of response to cyclosporin treatment for severe, steroid-resistant ulcerative colitis. *Am J Gastroenterol* 2000; 95: 2000-8.
21. Jarnerot G, Hertervig E, Friis-Liby I, *et al.* Infliximab as rescue therapy in severe to moderately severe ulcerative colitis: a randomized, placebo-controlled study. *Gastroenterology* 2005; 128: 1805-11.
22. Monterubbianesi R, Armuzzi A, Papi C, *et al.* Infliximab for severe ulcerative colitis: short-term and one-year outcome of three dose regimen. An Italian multicentre open-label study. *Gastroenterology* 2009; 138(Suppl 1): S685.
23. Venu M, Naik AS, Ananthakrishnan AN. Early infliximab infusion in hospitalised severe UC patients: one-year outcome. *Gastroenterology* 2009; 136(Suppl 1): A201.
24. Gustavsson A, Jarnerot G, Hertevig E, *et al.* Colectomy after rescue therapy in intravenous steroid-resistant acute ulcerative colitis: a 3-year follow-up study of the Swedish/Danish Infliximab/Placebo Trial. *Gut* 2008; 57: A79.
25. Jakobovits SL, Jewell DP, Travis SP. Infliximab for the treatment of ulcerative colitis: outcomes in Oxford from 2000 to 2006. *Aliment Pharmacol Ther* 2007; 25: 1055-60.
26. Kohn A, Daperno M, Armuzzi A, *et al.* Infliximab in severe ulcerative colitis: short-term results of different infusion regimens and long-term follow-up. *Aliment Pharmacol Ther* 2007; 26: 747-56.
27. Zisman TL, Lewis JR, Stein AC, *et al.* Predictors of avoidance of colectomy with infliximab initiation in severe, IV steroid-refractory ulcerative colitis. *Gastroenterology* 2009; 136(Suppl 1): A660.
28. Lees CW, Heys D, Ho GT, *et al.* A retrospective analysis of the efficacy and safety of infliximab as rescue therapy in acute severe ulcerative colitis. *Aliment Pharmacol Ther* 2007; 26: 411-9.
29. Laharie, BourellieA, Branche J, *et al.* Cyclosporine versus infliximab in acute severe ulcerative colitis refractory to intravenous steroids: a randomised study. *Gastroenterology* 2011; 139: 619.
30. Maser EA, Deconda D, Lichtiger S, *et al.* Cyclosporine and infliximab as acute salvage therapies for each other, in severe steroid-refractory ulcerative colitis. *Gut* 2007; 132: S1132.
31. Leblanc S, Allez M, Seksik P, *et al.* Successive treatment with cyclosporine and infliximab in severe ulcerative colitis. *Gastroenterology* 2009; 136(Suppl 1): A88.
32. Manosa M, Lopez San RA, Garcia-Planella E, *et al.* Infliximab rescue therapy after cyclosporin failure in steroid-refractory ulcerative colitis. *Digestion* 2009; 80: 30-5.
33. Sternthal MB, Murphy SJ, George J, *et al.* Adverse events associated with the use of cyclosporine in patients with inflammatory bowel disease. *Am J Gastroenterol* 2008; 103: 937-43.
34. Fidder H, Schnitzler F, Ferrante M, *et al.* Long-term safety of infliximab for the treatment of inflammatory bowel disease: a single-centre cohort study. *Gut* 2009; 58: 501-8.
35. Lichtenstein GR, Cohen RD, Feagan BG, *et al.* Safety of infliximab and other Crohn's disease therapies: Treat Registry data with 27,762 patient-year follow-up. *Gastroenterology* 2010; 138(Suppl 1): S475.

36. UK IBD Audit second round. http://www.rcplondon.ac.uk/clinical-standards/ceeu/Current-work/IBD/Pages/Overview.aspx.
37. Arnott IDR, Leiper K, Down C, *et al.* Outcome of acute severe ulcerative colitis: data from the national UK IBD Audit. *Gut* 2009; 58: A33.
38. Kaplan GG, McCarthy EP, Ayanian JZ, *et al.* Impact of hospital volume on postoperative morbidity and mortality following a colectomy for ulcerative colitis. *Gastroenterology* 2008; 134: 680-7.
39. Ananthakrishnan AN, McGinley EL, Binion DG. Inflammatory bowel disease in the elderly is associated with worse outcomes: a national study of hospitalizations. *Inflamm Bowel Dis* 2009; 15: 182-9.
40. Nguyen GC, Steinhart AH. Nationwide patterns of hospitalizations to centers with high volume of admissions for inflammatory bowel disease and their impact on mortality. *Inflamm Bowel Dis* 2008; 14: 1688-94.
41. Roberts SE, Williams JG, Yeates D, *et al.* Mortality in patients with and without colectomy admitted to hospital for ulcerative colitis and Crohn's disease: record linkage studies. *BMJ* 2007; 335: 1033.
42. Nicholls RJ, Clark DN, Kelso L, *et al.* Nationwide linkage analysis in Scotland implicates age as the critical overall determinant of mortality in ulcerative colitis. *Aliment Pharmacol Ther* 2010; 31: 1310-21.
43. Randall J, Singh B, Warren BF, *et al.* Delayed surgery for acute severe colitis is associated with increased risk of postoperative complications. *Br J Surg* 2010; 97: 404-9.
44. Yang Z, Wu Q, Wu K, *et al.* Meta-analysis: pre-operative infliximab treatment and short-term post-operative complications in patients with ulcerative colitis. *Aliment Pharmacol Ther* 2010; 31: 486-92.
45. Andersson P, Soderholm JD. Surgery in ulcerative colitis: indication and timing. *Dig Dis* 2009; 27: 335-40.

Chapter 5

Surgery in ulcerative colitis

Janindra Warusavitarne BMed PhD FRACS Consultant Colorectal Surgeon, St Mark's Hospital, London, UK
Josef Watfah MD Surgical Registrar, St Mark's Hospital, London, UK

Overview

Despite advances in medical treatment for ulcerative colitis (UC), 25-30% will require surgery at some time during their life. Emergency surgery is required in patients with toxic megacolon or perforation and elective surgery is indicated in patients who have failed medical therapy or have a high risk of malignancy. Restorative proctocolectomy (RPC) with ileal pouch-anal anastomosis (IPAA) introduced by Sir Alan Parks and John Nicholls in 1976 [1] has revolutionised surgical treatment for UC. Before this the treatment of choice was proctocolectomy with formation of an end ileostomy. A multidisciplinary approach is needed between the surgeon, gastroenterologist, stoma therapist and specialist nurse to ensure optimal outcomes. The patient needs to be actively involved in the decision-making process.

Introduction

The decision to perform surgery in ulcerative colitis (UC) should be ideally made in a multidisciplinary team setting. As a general rule, surgery is the appropriate choice of treatment where medical treatment options have failed (chronic refractory), where there is an imminent risk of perforation (acute), or the risk of malignancy is high [2] (Table 1).

Table 1. Indications for surgery.

Acute	Chronic	Risk of malignancy
Toxic megacolon	Refractory to medical treatment	High-grade dyplastic polyps (DALMs) – not endoscopically treatable
Perforation	Inability to wean off long-term steroid treatment	Adequate endoscopic surveillance not possible

Surgical options

The two main options for surgical treatment for UC are panproctocolectomy with formation of an end ileostomy or restorative proctocolectomy (RPC) with an ileal pouch-anal anastomosis (IPAA). In some circumstances, a further option is a total colectomy with an ileorectal anastomosis.

Panproctocolectomy with end ileostomy

This operation involves removal of the colon and rectum and results in a permanent end ileostomy. Suitable patients for this operation may include patients with incontinence and poor sphincter function prior to the operation; relevant comorbidity; a low rectal tumour when margins might be compromised; patient's decision (having discussed the advantages and disadvantages of the different options); patients with a history of perianal disease (fissure, fistula or abscess).

Restorative proctocolectomy (RPC) with ileal pouch-anal anastomosis (IPAA)

This operation can be done as a one-, two- or three-stage procedure. A one-stage procedure involves a panproctocolectomy and formation of an ileoanal pouch without a covering loop ileostomy. A two-stage procedure involves a panproctocolectomy and formation of an ileoanal pouch with a defunctioning loop ileostomy and, in the second stage, closure of the loop ileostomy. A three-stage procedure involves a subtotal colectomy with end ileostomy, followed by a completion proctectomy and formation of an ileoanal pouch with a temporary covering loop ileostomy and, in the third stage, closure of the loop ileostomy.

Pouch surgery appears to be the preferred choice for most patients. Although age is not a contraindication to pouch surgery, patients older than 60 years may experience poor functional results [3]. It is important to obtain a detailed history of sphincter function and perform anorectal physiology and endoanal ultrasound in this group of patients in order to counsel them about the risk of incontinence after pouch surgery. The ileoanal pouch procedure is also associated with a 40% reduction of fecundity. This risk should be foremost in any discussion with a woman of child-bearing age. The option to delay the second stage of surgery should form part of this discussion to minimise the effect on fecundity.

In approximately 15% of patients with colitis, the diagnosis of indeterminate colitis is made. Indeterminate colitis is not an absolute contraindication but the rate of pelvic sepsis and pouch failure is increased by approximately 16% [4, 5]. This should be discussed in pre-operative counselling.

Total colectomy and ileorectal anastomosis

This procedure has very limited indications. The main benefit of this procedure is that it allows retention of the rectum which results in better function with minimal effects on fecunditiy and erectile dysfunction. A nona

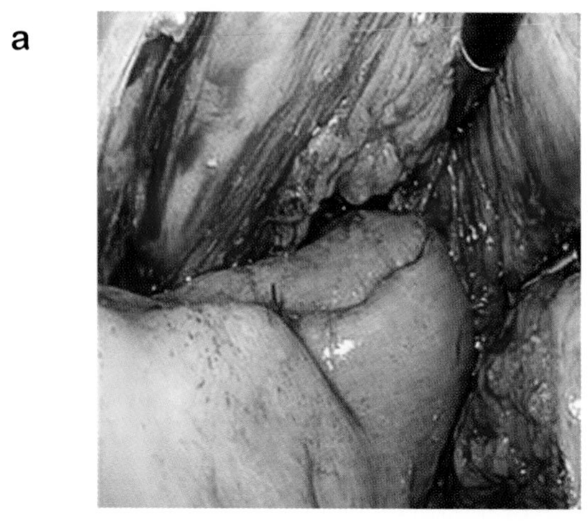

b

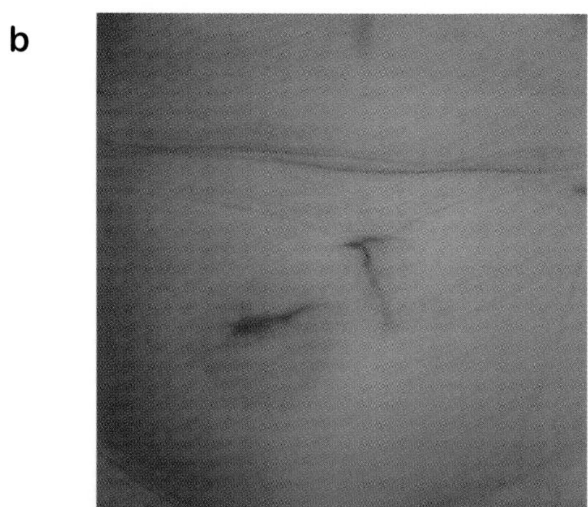

Figure 1. a) Laparoscopic view of ileoanal pouch anastomosis. b) Abdominal incisions after laparoscopic surgery (includes stoma closure site).

inflamed rectum is essential for the success of this procedure, limiting the number of patients suitable for the procedure. The risk of proctitis after the procedure is not well known as this procedure is not commonly performed. Any discussion with the patient should mention this risk and the effect of proctitis on function. Surveillance of the rectal remnant should be performed and this does not preclude the patient from having a RPC in the future.

Surgical approach

The traditional approach to surgery for UC has been by laparotomy (Figure 1). Recent advances in laparoscopy and laparoscopic experience has made this approach feasible in surgery for UC. The advantages of laparoscopy in surgery for UC are shorter fasting time, a shorter postoperative stay and better cosmesis. A recent meta-analysis has shown a lower overall complication rate [6] than open surgery.

The outcomes of pouch surgery are related to the volume of surgical procedures performed. High-volume centres tend to have better outcomes independent of surgical approach (open or laparoscopic).

Pouch formation

In the original operation described by Parks and Nicholls, an 'S' configuration was used. Other configurations such as the J, W and K pouches have been described. The J pouch is the most commonly performed pouch [7] and is typically 15-20cm in length. Shorter pouches result in increased frequency and longer pouches have emptying difficulties.

The anastomosis can either be double-stapled or handsewn. The double-stapled anastomosis tends to be the preferred and the most commonly performed option, where a stapling device transects the rectum leaving no more than a 1-2cm cuff of the anal transitional zone and the pouch anal anstomosis is performed with a circular stapling device. A technical failure with the stapling device can be encountered occasionally and the surgeon should be adequately trained in the handsewn technique. The handsewn technique is also indicated in situations where all the rectal mucosa and the transitional epithelium needs to be excised such as in the care of dysplasia or transitional zone inflammation. The handsewn technique is associated with a higher risk of mucus leak and faecal seepage as the anal transitional zone has been excised.

Pouch function

An individual with an ileoanal pouch empties the pouch on average 4-5 times a day and approximately once at night. The frequency of pouch emptying can increase with changes in diet and dietary counselling should be offered to patients before and after surgery. A pouch support nurse can be a valuable resource in any institution and can provide clinical support and lifestyle information.

Complications

Surgery for UC is associated with a very low mortality (<1%) as most patients are young at presentation for surgery. The morbidity for RPC is high (>20%) and can be divided into early and late complications (Table 2).

Table 2. Early/acute and late/chronic complications of RPC.

Early/acute complications	Late/chronic complications
Anastomotic leak	Pouchitis
Haemorrhage from the pouch	Cuffitis
Small bowel obstruction	Pouch fistula
Pelvic sepsis (suture line leaks, bacterial contamination, infected pelvic haematoma)	Pouch stricture
	Sexual dysfunction
	Chronic pelvis sepsis
	Pouch failure

Early/acute complications

Early recognition and prompt treatment is important to minimise long-term pouch failure and poor function. Digital rectal examination may reveal an anastomotic defect, but CT or MRI may be more reliable. Treatment with antibiotics or radiological drainage may solve minor septic complications, but if the sepsis persists an EUA should be performed and any collection can be drained through the pouch anal anastomosis. If the patient deteriorates with signs of peritonism, laparotomy or laparoscopy should be performed. It may be necessary to perform a defunctioning ileostomy if one is not present at this time. In extreme circumstances disconnection of the pouch may be necessary. Bleeding from the pouch may occur at a staple of the suture line and can be controlled locally in most situations [8].

The risk of small bowel obstruction (SBO) after pouch surgery ranges from 15-44% and can occur at any time after surgery. In most situations resolution occurs with conservative treatment. The commonest sites of obstruction are the pelvis and site of ileostomy closure [9]. Surgery for SBO should be avoided from day 14 after surgery until 3 months owing to dense adhesions which can result in enterotomies and enterocutaneous fistula formation.

Late/chronic complications

Pouchitis is the most common chronic complication of pouch surgery. The incidence of pouchitis in patients having a pouch for UC is estimated at 30-50% with the incidence increasing to 80% in the presence of primary sclerosing cholangitis. The aetiology of pouchitis is unknown but it is thought to be related to the host response to bacterial colonisation in the pouch. The diagnosis is made on clinical, endoscopic and histological features. Treatment includes ciprofloxacin and metronidazole and symptomatic therapy. The probiotic VSL#3 has been shown to be effective as maintainance therapy after inducing remission with antibiotics. The relapse rate with VSL#3 maintenance is 10-15% compared with 94-100% for placebo[10]. In approximately 10% of patients, pouchitis does not respond to antibiotic treatment and defunctioning the pouch may be necessary. For a detailed description on the management of pouchitis, see Chapter 6.

Cuffitis (inflammation of the remnant cuff) occurs in about 20% of patients and can be successfully treated with steroid suppositories or enemas.

Pouch fistulae are more often seen as a late complication. Pouch vaginal or pouch perineal fistulae occur in 5-10% of patients with UC. Where the diagnosis of Crohn's disease is made after the colectomy, pouch vaginal or pouch perineal fistulae occur in about 25% of patients. Placing a seton is the treatment of choice as fistulotomy may result in incontinence. In some circumstances it may be necessary to re-do the pouch or defunction the pouch permanently if there is no symptomatic control with a seton.

An anastomotic stricture can be treated with dilatation which can be performed by the patient at home after initial dilatation under anaesthesia.

The risk of pouch failure increases with time and the commonest reasons for failure which result in a permanent ileostomy are refractory pouchitis and pelvic sepsis. The overall risk of pouch failure is 9% over 10 years and risk assesment can be carried out by using such models as the the Cleveland Clinic Foundation ileal pouch failure model [11].

Re-do pouch surgery

Re-do pouch surgery is very challenging and can be associated with significant morbidity. Results from specialist centres for pouch surgery in North America, Germany and UK have shown high success rates and good functional outcomes for re-do reconstructive pouch surgery performed by experienced surgeons.

New techniques and future outlook

Single-port laparoscopic surgery (SPLS) has been performed for pouch surgery, using the stoma site as the only access site for surgery. Despite good outcomes in selected patients, the only benefit is superior cosmesis [12].

Conclusions

The decision to perform surgery in UC is one that requires multidisciplinary input. High-volume centres appear to have better results in pouch surgery. The laparoscopic approach to pouch surgery in experienced hands should be considered as the first-line option.

Key points

- Treatment of UC needs a multidisciplinary team approach.
- Surgery is an important part of the treatment of patients with UC.
- Emergency surgery is indicated in patients with acute toxic megacolon or perforation.
- Elective surgery is indicated when medical treatment has failed or the risk of malignancy is high.
- Restorative proctocolectomy is the surgical procedure of choice with an increased percentage of operations being performed laparoscopically.
- Contraindications for pouch surgery are poor sphincter function, a low rectal tumour with the risk of compromising margins and patient choice.
- Morbidity for pouch surgery is around 20% and patients must be counselled appropriately.
- Surgeons and gastroenterologists must be aware of complications and treat them as a team to optimise the outcome for patients.
- An average of 10% of pouches fail after 10 years.
- Re-do pouch surgery can be considered in selected cases and should be performed in specialist centres.

References

1. Parks AG, Nicholls RJ. Proctocolectomy without ileostomy for ulcerative colitis. *Br Med J* 1978, 2: 85-8.
2. Eaden JA, Abrams KR, Mayberry JF. The risk of colorectal cancer in ulcerative colitis: a meta-analysis. *Gut* 2001; 48: 526-35.
3. Delaney CP, Dadvand B, Remzi FH, *et al.* Functional outcome, quality of life and complications after ileal pouch-anal anastomosis in selected septuagenarians. *Colon Rectum* 2002; 45: 890-4.
4. Mc Intyre PB, Pemberton JH, Wolff BG, *et al.* Indeterminate colitis. Long-term outcome in patients after ileal pouch-anal anastomosis. *Dis Colon Rectum* 1995; 38: 51-4.
5. Tekkis PP, Heriot AG, Smith O, *et al.* Long-term outcomes of restorative proctocolectomy for Crohn's disease and indeterminate colitis. *Colorectal Dis* 2005; 7: 218-23.
6. Xiao-Jian W, Xiao-Sheng H, Xu-Yu Z, *et al.* The role of laparoscopic surgery for ulcerative colitis: systematic review with meta-analysis. *Int J Colorectal Dis* 2010; 25: 949-57.
7. Utsunomiya J, Iwana T, Imajo M, *et al.* Total colectomy, mucosal proctectomy and ileoanal anastomosis. *Dis Colon Rectum* 1980, 23: 459-66.
8. Fazio VW, Ziv Y, Church JM. Ileal pouch-anal anastomosis complications and function in 1005 patients. *Ann Surg* 2002; 222: 120-7.
9. Mac Lean AR, Cohen Z, Mac Rae HM, *et al.* Risk of small bowel obstruction after ileal-pouch anastomosis. *Ann Surg* 2002; 235: 200-6.
10. Gionchetti P, Rizzello F, Helwig U, *et al.* Prophylaxis of pouchitis onset with probiotic therapy. A double-blind placebo controlled trial. *Gastroenterology* 2003; 124: 1202-9.
11. Fazio VW, Tekkis PP, Remzi F, *et al.* Quantification of risk for pouch failure after ileal pouch-anal anastomosis surgery. *Ann Surg* 2003; 238: 605-17.
12. Geisler DP, Kirat HT, Remzi FH. Single-port laparoscopic total proctectomy with ileal pouch-anal anastomosis: initial operative experience. *Surg Endosc* 2011; 25: 2175-8.

Chapter 6

Management of pouchitis

Jonathan Landy MRCP Research Fellow and Specialist Registrar, St Mark's Hospital, London, UK
Susan K. Clark MA MB BChir MD FRCS(Gen Surg) Consultant Colorectal Surgeon, St Mark's Hospital, London, UK

Overview

Restorative proctocoloectomy is the procedure of choice for patients with ulcerative colitis (UC) undergoing colectomy. Over 6000 patients in the UK have undergone restorative proctocolectomy, and gastroenterologists as well as surgeons are increasingly involved in their long-term management.

Pouchitis is the most common cause of pouch dysfunction. This is usually responsive to antibiotics and only 10-15% of patients suffer chronic pouchitis. Other causes of pouch dysfunction and inflammation should be considered and excluded before making a diagnosis of pouchitis. Pouchoscopy and biopsy should be undertaken before treatment is initiated. The mainstay of treatment is antibiotics.

We discuss the epidemiology, risk factors, diagnosis of pouchitis and the differential diagnoses to consider. We review the evidence for the treatment of pouchitis including alternative therapies for pouchitis that is refractory to antibiotics and suggest a management algorithm for these patients.

Introduction

Up to 35% [1] of patients with ulcerative colitis (UC) eventually require surgery. For the majority of patients, restorative proctocolectomy with ileal pouch-anal anastomosis (RPC and IPAA) is the operation of choice [2]. It is also used for some patients with familial adenomatous polyposis (FAP). The procedure involves the removal of the colon and rectum and the construction of a reservoir (pouch) created from 30-40cm of ileum, followed by ileoanal anastomosis [3]. This procedure avoids the need for a permanent stoma and can allow good long-term function and quality of life that is comparable to the general population [4]. Over 6000 patients in the UK have undergone restorative proctocolectomy.

Pouch failure has been defined as the need for removal of the pouch and the establishment of a permanent ileostomy or the need for an ileostomy without prospect of closure. Failure rates increase with time and after 20 years around 10-15% of patients require the establishment of a permanent ileostomy. The majority of pouch failures (50%) are due to pelvic sepsis.

Poor function accounts for up to 30% of pouch failure [5]. This may be due to mechanical outlet obstruction due to stricture formation, or functional abnormalities such as sphincter weakness, a small-volume pouch or irritable pouch syndrome, where there is no apparent cause of pouch dysfunction.

Other systemic and gastrointestinal pathologies can cause high pouch output such as hyperthyroidism, coeliac disease, lactose intolerance, pancreatic insufficiency, bacterial overgrowth and bile salt malabsorption. Pouchitis is the most common cause of pouch dysfunction and accounts for 10-15% of pouch failures [5].

Pouchitis

Pouchitis is an idiopathic inflammatory condition that may occur in up to 50% of patients after RPC for ulcerative colitis. It is rarely seen in FAP patients after RPC. The incidence of pouchitis increases with longer follow-up. Up to 60% of patients may suffer a recurrence, but the prevalence of chronic pouchitis is only 5-10% [6].

A number of risk factors for pouchitis have been reported. Extensive or severe UC, backwash ileitis, extraintestinal manifestations, pre-colectomy thrombocytosis, pANCA positivity and non-steroidal use have all been reported as risk factors for the development of pouchitis, although they have not been demonstrated consistently [7]. Primary sclerosing cholangitis is associated with a two-fold increase in risk of pouchitis [8].

The aetiology of pouchitis remains unknown. An overlap with ulcerative colitis is suggested by the frequency with which it affects patients with UC compared with FAP. Genetic factors including a CARD 15 polymorphism have been shown to be exclusive to chronic pouchitis [7]. The characteristic resolution of acute pouchitis with antibiotic treatment strongly implicates bacteria. Pouchitis does not occur until after the diverting ileostomy is closed and the faecal stream flows through the pouch leading to a vast increase in the bacterial flora within the pouch. A number of studies suggest a dysbiosis in pouchitis [9]. Abnormalities of epithelial barrier function and the host immune response are also likely to be significant factors in the underlying pathogenesis of pouchitis.

Clinical characteristics of pouchitis

The diagnosis of pouchitis requires the combination of clinical symptoms as well as endoscopic and histological findings. Clinical symptoms include increased stool frequency and liquidity, abdominal cramping, urgency and tenesmus, and occasionally rectal bleeding and fever. Endoscopic assessment and biopsy with flexible pouchoscopy should be undertaken (Figure 1). Symptoms do not always correlate with endoscopic and histological findings. A number of pouchitis scoring systems are in use. The Pouch Disease Activity Index (PDAI) (Table 1) is commonly used.

Pouchitis can be classified according to disease activity, duration, pattern and response to antibiotics. Acute pouchitis can be considered as

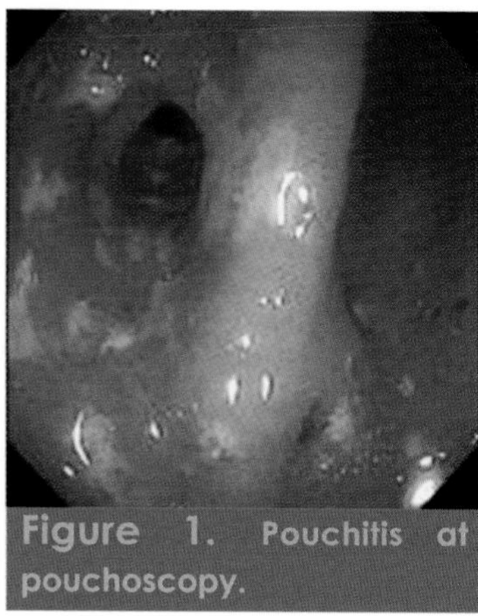

Figure 1. Pouchitis at pouchoscopy.

less than 4 weeks' duration, responding to a single antibiotic and occurring less than three times per year. Chronic pouchitis may be considered to be chronic relapsing if there are three or more episodes per year responding to antibiotics or chronic antibiotic-dependent if symptoms are only controlled while maintained on antibiotics. Chronic antibiotic-refractory pouchitis is generally defined as pouchitis that no longer responds to a single antibiotic.

Differential diagnoses

Inflammation of the pouch can also occur for a number of other reasons that should be considered in the differential diagnosis of pouchitis. Pelvic sepsis can cause the clinical, endoscopic and histological findings of pouchitis and partially responds to antibiotic treatment. A history of early postoperative complications or fistula may be suggestive and MRI should be performed where pelvic sepsis is suspected.

Pre-pouch ileitis is inflammation developing in the ileum immediately proximal to the pouch. It is usually concurrent with pouchitis, but can occur in isolation. Symptoms include those of pouchitis, but may also include those of intestinal obstruction. A number of treatments for pre-pouch ileitis

Table 1. Pouch Disease Activity Index.

Criteria	Score
Clinical	
Stool frequency	
Usual postoperative stool frequency	0
1-2 stools/day > postoperative usual	1
≥3 stools/day > postoperative usual	2
Rectal bleeding	
None or rare	0
Present daily	1
Faecal urgency or abdominal cramps	
None	0
Occasional	1
Usual	2
Fever (temperature >37.8°C)	
Absent	0
Present	1
Endoscopic inflammation	
Oedema	1
Granularity	1
Friability	1
Loss of vascular pattern	1
Mucous exudate	1
Ulceration	1
Acute histological inflammation	
Polymorphonuclear leucocyte infiltration	
Mild	1
Moderate + crypt abscess	2
Severe + crypt abscess	3
Ulceration per lower power field (mean)	
<25%	1
25-50%	2
>50%	3

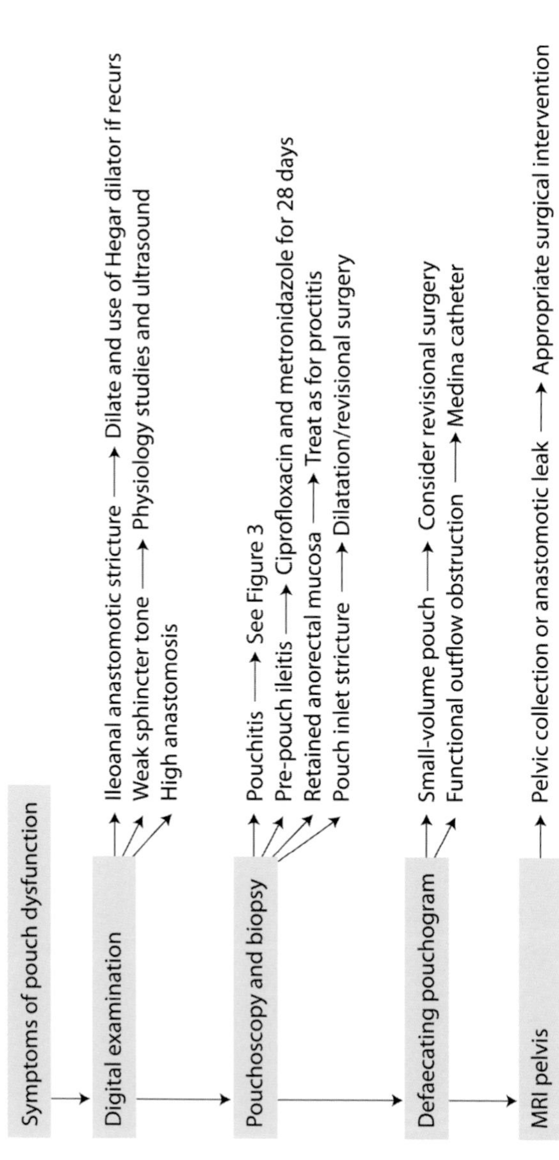

Figure 2. Algorithm for investigation of pouch dysfunction.

have been described including steroids, antibiotics and 5-ASA medications [10].

Inflammation of the remaining anorectal mucosa (cuffitis) can also be a cause of symptoms similar to pouchitis with endoscopic inflammation. Persisting proctitis of residual anorectal mucosa may lead to bleeding, urgency, and frequency of small-volume stool. The presence of inflamed rectal mucosa will be confirmed on biopsy. Treatment is with 5-ASA or steroid suppositories or in severe persistent cases revision of the anastomosis may be undertaken.

Two to three percent of patients diagnosed with ulcerative colitis pre-operatively are subsequently found to have Crohn's disease. Crohn's disease should be considered where there is fistulation or chronic unremitting pouchitis. Cytomegalovirus and *Clostridium difficile* may cause pouch inflammation. Both are uncommon, but should be excluded in recurrent or refractory pouchitis. Figure 2 shows an algorithm for investigation of pouch dysfunction.

Treatment of pouchitis

Antibiotics

Antibiotics are the mainstay of treatment for pouchitis. The majority of patients will respond to a course of a single agent or combination of antibiotics and remain in remission. Both ciprofloxacin and metronidazole for 14 days have been shown to be effective as first-line therapy for pouchitis. For the treatment of acute pouchitis ciprofloxacin has been shown to be more effective and better tolerated than metronidazole. For patients in whom ciprofloxacin is ineffective and who are intolerant of oral metronidazole, topical metronidazole may be of benefit. In a randomised controlled trial of rifaximin, 25% in the rifaximin group compared with none in the placebo group achieved remission [11].

Patients who fail to respond to a single antibiotic or have early relapse, may respond to combination therapy with two antibiotics. Combination therapy using rifaximin and ciprofloxacin for 15 days [12] and ciprofloxacin and metronidazole or tinidazole for 4 weeks [13, 14] were shown to achieve remission in up to 80% of patients. Patients with chronic pouchitis who achieve remission following antibiotic therapy, but relapse more than three times per year should be treated with maintenance therapy. Maintenance with metronidazole at doses ranging from 250mg every 3 days to 750mg daily may be effective. However, adverse effects may occur. Consequently, ciprofloxacin is often used to maintain remission in patients with chronic antibiotic-dependent pouchitis and can be used at less than full doses, although there are no long-term data.

Long-term treatment with ciprofloxacin may lead to the development of antibiotic resistance and extended spectrum beta-lactamase-producing (ESBL) bacteria. A prospective study of faecal samples from 48 patients with chronic pouchitis identified ESBL-producing organisms in a third of patients [15]. A further study of chronic pouchitis patients with antibiotic resistance demonstrated that faecal coliform sensitivity analysis could identify effective antibiotic therapies for patients with an 80% remission rate using a targeted antibiotic approach [16].

Probiotics

The probiotic VSL#3 has been shown to be effective in maintenance of remission of pouchitis. Two randomised, double-blind placebo-controlled studies of VSL#3 (containing 5×10^{11} per gram of viable lyophilized bacteria of four strains of Lactobacilli, three strains of Bifidobacteria, and 1 strain of *Streptococcus salivarius* subsp. *Thermophilus*) to maintain remission in chronic pouchitis have been undertaken [11]. Following induction of remission with open-label ciprofloxacin and rifaximin, or ciprofloxacin and metronidazole, relapse rates were 15% for the VSL#3 group compared with 100% for placebo group [11].

Two studies investigated the efficacy of oral probiotic therapy with VSL#3 in the prevention of pouchitis. In a randomised trial of VSL#3, initiated within 1 week of ileostomy closure after IPAA, 20% of the VSL#3 group and 40% of the placebo group had an episode of pouchitis at 1 year [17]. However, in another study, no significant difference between VSL#3 and no treatment was found [18].

For patients with chronic pouchitis, maintenance therapy with VSL#3 has been recommended in the current British Society of Gastroenterology IBD guidelines [19]. However, subsequent clinical studies have reported disappointing results with less than 20% of patients maintaining remission [20]. The studies finding VSL#3 to be effective were limited by the exclusion of patients who did not achieve complete or near complete mucosal healing with antibiotic induction therapy. A significant proportion of pouchitis patients are consequently unlikely to benefit from treatment with probiotics.

Other treatments

A number of other therapies for pouchitis have been reported in uncontrolled studies. Oral and topical steroids may be of benefit. Two small open-label studies of oral budesonide showed a 75-80% remission rate in patients with chronic pouchitis unresponsive to antibiotics, treated with 9mg of budesonide for 8 weeks. A randomised, double-blind, double-dummy, placebo-controlled trial of budesonide enemas compared to metronidazole for acute pouchitis showed a 50% remission rate in the budesonide group compared with 43% in the metronidazole group [11]. There are no controlled trials of 5-ASA therapy for pouchitis. A study of combination ciprofloxacin and tinidazole for chronic refractory pouchitis compared outcome to a historic cohort treated with oral or topical mesalamine. For the mesalamine group there was a 50% clinical response and remission rate. A recently published pilot study of sulfasalazine (3g/day) in 11 patients with acute pouchitis demonstrated a 73% response and 63% remission rate with no adverse events [21]. As an alternative to long-term steroid use, thiopurines are sometimes used. Cyclosporine enemas have also been reported to be of benefit and infliximab was shown to be of benefit for patients with chronic pouchitis and ileitis or pouch anal fistulae.

A number of enema formulations have been considered. Two studies examined the role of bismuth carbomer enemas for chronic pouchitis. In an open-label study of 12 patients with chronic pouchitis, treated with bismuth carbomer enemas every third day over 45 days, 83% went into remission. Sixty percent remained in remission over 12 months with

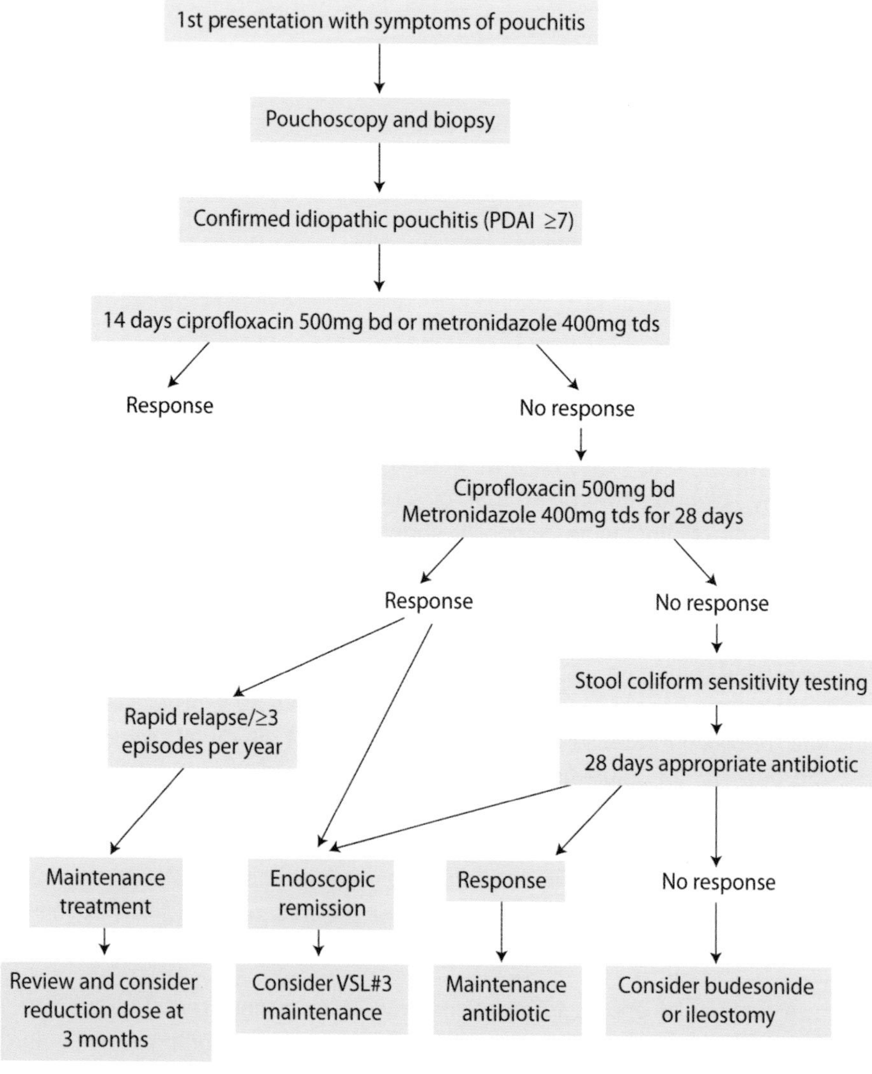
1st presentation with symptoms of pouchitis
Pouchoscopy and biopsy
Confirmed idiopathic pouchitis (PDAI ≥7)
14 days ciprofloxacin 500mg bd or metronidazole 400mg tds
Response
No response
Ciprofloxacin 500mg bd
Metronidazole 400mg tds for 28 days
Response
No response
Stool coliform sensitivity testing
Rapid relapse/≥3
episodes per year
28 days appropriate antibiotic
Maintenance
treatment
Endoscopic
remission
Response
No response
Review and consider
reduction dose at
3 months
Consider VSL#3
maintenance
Maintenance
antibiotic
Consider budesonide
or ileostomy

Figure 3. Algorithm of pouchitis management.

ongoing treatment. However, Tremaine *et al* treated 20 patients with bismuth carbomer foam enemas and 20 patients with dummy enemas for 3 weeks. There was no difference between treatment and placebo group in response to treatment [11]. A study of nine patients with chronic pouchitis treated with butyrate suppositories and 10 patients treated with glutamine suppositories for 21 days showed a 60% remission rate for glutamine versus a 33% remission rate for butyrate [11]. In an open-label uncontrolled study, 12 patients with chronic unremitting pouchitis were treated with an antisense inhibitor of intercellular adhesion molecule-1 (240mg alicaforsen enema, 60ml) nightly for 6 weeks. By week 6, 58% were in remission and 10 of the 12 patients had achieved a mucosal appearance score of 0 or 1 on pouchoscopy [22].

Conclusions

There are a number of causes of pouch dysfunction other than pouchitis. These should be excluded. Pouchoscopy and biopsy should be undertaken for the diagnosis of pouchitis. Most patients will respond to a single antibiotic, and either ciprofloxacin or metronidazole for 14 days can be used in the first instance. Up to 60% of patients may experience a recurrence and 5-10% may suffer chronic pouchitis. For initial non-responders to a single antibiotic, combination therapy should be given for 28 days. For those requiring long-term treatment, faecal sensitivity testing should be undertaken to exclude resistant organisms and targeted antibiotic therapy instigated accordingly. Long-term therapy with ciprofloxacin is better tolerated than metrondiazole. Reduced doses can be used for maintenance therapy. Following induction of remission with antibiotics, maintenance therapy with VSL#3 (6g/d) could be considered. For those patients who are unresponsive, budesonide could be considered. Other options including sulfasalazine, bismuth carbomer, immunomodulators or anti-TNF therapies have little evidence for their use. A small minority of patients will not respond to medical therapy and should be considered for permanent ileostomy with exclusion or excision of the pouch.

Figure 3 outlines an algorithm for pouchitis management.

Key points

- **Pouchitis occurs in up to 50% of patients undergoing RPC for UC, but chronic pouchitis occurs in only 10%.**
- **Other causes of pouch dysfunction and inflammation should be excluded.**
- **Antibiotics are the mainstay of treatment for pouchitis.**
- **Stool coliform sensitivity testing should be undertaken in patients unresponsive to antibiotics for targeted antibiotic therapy.**

References

1. Langholz E, Munkholm P, Davidsen M, Binder V. Long-term prognosis of patients with ulcerative colitis. *Ugeskr Laeger* 1993; 155(46): 3767-72.
2. Becker JM. Surgical management of inflammatory bowel disease. *Curr Opinion Gastroenterol* 1993; 9: 600-15.
3. Parks AG, Nicholls RJ. Proctocolectomy without ileostomy for ulcerative colitis. *Br Med J* 1978; 2(6130): 85-8.
4. Carmon E, Keider A, Ravid A *et al.* The correlation between quality of life and functional outcome in ulcerative colitis patients after proctocolectomy ileal pouch anal anastomosis. *Colorectal Dis* 2003; 5: 228-32.
5. Tulchinsky H, Hawley P, Nicholls J. Long-term failure after restorative proctocolectomy for ulcerative colitis. *Ann Surg* 2003; 238: 229-34.
6. Simchuk EJ, Thirlby RC. Risk factors and true incidence of pouchitis in patients after ileal pouch-anal anastomoses. *World J Surg* 2000; 24: 851-6.
7. Pardi DS, Sandborn WJ. Systemic review: the management of pouchitis. *Aliment Pharmacol Ther* 2006; 23: 1087-96.
8. Zins BJ, Sandborn WJ, Penna CR, *et al.* Pouchitis disease course after orthotopic liver transplantation in patients with ulcerative colitis and primary sclerosing cholangitis and an ileal pouch-anal anastomosis. *Am J Gastroenterol* 1995; 90: 2177-81.
9. McLaughlin SD, Walker AW, Churcher C, *et al.* The bacteriology of pouchitis. A molecular phylogenetic analysis using 16S rRNA gene cloning and sequencing. *Ann Surg* 2010; 252: 90-8.
10. McLaughlin SD, Clark SK, Bell AJ, *et al.* An open study of antibiotics for the treatment for pre-pouch ileitis following restorative proctocolectomy with ileal-pouch anal anastomosis: efficacy, complications and outcomes. *Colorectal Dis* 2011; 13: 438-44.
11. Holubar S, Cima R, Sandborn WJ, Pardi DS. Treatment and prevention of pouchitis after ileal pouch-anal anstomosis for chronic ulcerative colitis (Review). *Cochrane Database Syst Rev* 2010; 6: CD001176.

12. Abdelrazeq AS, Kelly SM, Lund JN, Leveson SH. Rifaximin-ciprofloxacin combination therapy is effective in chronic active refractory pouchitis. *Colorectal Dis* 2005; 7: 182-6.
13. Mimura T, Rizello F, Helwig U, *et al.* Four-week open label trial of metronidazole and ciprofloxacin for the treatment of recurrent or refractory pouchitis. *Aliment Pharmacol Ther* 2002; 16: 909-17.
14. Shen B, Fazio VW, Remzi FH, *et al.* Combined ciprofloxacin and tinidazole therapy in the treatment of chronic refractory pouchitis. *Dis Colon Rectum* 2007; 50: 498-508.
15. McLaughlin SD, Clark SK, Roberts CH, *et al.* Extended spectrum beta-lactamase-producing bacteria and *Clostridium difficile* in patients with pouchitis. *Aliment Pharmacol Ther* 2010; 32: 664-9.
16. McLaughlin SD, Clark SK, Shafi S, *et al.* Fecal coliform testing to identify effective antibiotic therapies for patients with antibiotic-resistant pouchitis. *Clin Gastroenterol Hepatol* 2009; 7: 545-8.
17. Gionchetti P, Rizello F, Helwig U. Prophylaxis of pouchitis onset with probiotic therapy: a double-blind, placebo-controlled pilot study. *Inflamm Bowel Dis* 2007; 13(10): 1250-5.
18. Pronio A, Montesani C, Butteroni C, *et al.* Probiotic administration in patients with ileal pouch-anal anastomosis for ulcerative colitis is associated with expansion of mucosal regulatory cells. *Inflamm Bowel Dis* 2008; 14: 662-8.
19. Carter MJ, Lobo AJ, Travis SP. Guidelines for the management of inflammatory bowel disease in adults. *Gut* 2004; 53 Suppl 5: V1-16.
20. Shen B, Brzezinski A, Fazio VW, *et al.* Maintenance therapy with a probiotic in antibiotic-dependent pouchitis: experience in clinical practice. *Aliment Pharmacol Ther* 2005; 22: 721-8.
21. Belluzzi A, Serrani M, Roda G, *et al.* Pilot study: the use of sulfasalazine for the treatment of acute pouchitis. *Aliment Pharmacol Ther* 2010; 31: 228-32.
22. Miner P, Wedel M, Bane B, Bradley S. An enema formulation of alicaforsen, an antisense inhibitor of intercellular adhesion molecule-1, in the treatment of chronic, unremitting pouchitis. *Aliment Pharmacol Ther* 2004; 19: 281-6.

Part 2 Introduction

Management of Crohn's disease

Siew Ng MBBS PhD MRCP Assistant Professor, Institute of Digestive Disease, Department of Medicine and Therapeutics, Chinese University of Hong Kong, Hong Kong; Senior Lecturer and Honorary Gastroenterologist, St Vincent's Hospital, University of Melbourne, Australia

Crohn's disease is a chronic inflammatory bowel disease of unknown aetiology affecting any part of the gastrointestinal tract from the mouth to the anus. It commonly affects the ileum, colon and perineum, and is characterised by transmural granulomatous inflammation. Crohn's disease is incurable; it begins in young adulthood and continues throughout life. Afflicting mostly young people at an age when they are most active both in their professional and private life, Crohn's disease not only affects patients physically but also psychologically and socially.

The hallmarks of Crohn's disease include abdominal pain, diarrhoea, weight loss, rectal bleeding and fever. Upper gastrointestinal and jejuno-ileal disease are more common in adolescents compared with adults in whom colonic disease is more common. Perianal fistulae occur in around a third of patients and can be debilitating. The Montreal classification for Crohn's disease takes into account the age of diagosis, location and behaviour of disease (Table 1) [1].

Table 1. Montreal classification of Crohn's disease [1].

Age at diagnosis	Location	Behaviour
A1 <16 years	L1 ileal	B1 inflammatory
A2 17-40 years	L2 colonic	B2 stricturing
A3 >40 years	L3 ileo-colonic	B3 penetrating
	*L4 isolated upper GI disease	†p perianal disease

*L4 is a modifier that can be added to L1-L3
†p is a modifier that can be added to B1-B3

The natural history of Crohn's disease is now better appreciated. In the first year after diagnosis, 50% of all Crohn's patients will experience a flare of disease, irrespective of the site of disease. Of these, about one-third will have a single flare and two-thirds will have at least two relapses. Over time most patients with Crohn's disease progress from inflammatory to stricturing or penetrating complications. In contrast to those with ileal disease, patients with Crohn's colitis mostly remain uncomplicated over many years. Lesions usually arise from a single intestinal segment and disease site tends to be stable over time.

Despite advances in medical therapy, three-quarters of patients with Crohn's disease require an operation in their lifetime, and surgery is not curative. Surgery is reserved for complications of disease, or for severe limited disease unresponsive to medical therapy. Similar to that of ulcerative colitis, the goals of treatment in Crohn's disease should extend beyond symptomatic remission to include improvement in quality of life and mucosal healing; the latter endpoint has been shown to predict long-term outcome and is associated with less clinical relapse, a decreased need for hospitalisation and less need for surgery. In the clinical trial setting, disease activity in Crohn's disease has been defined most commonly by the Crohn's Disease Activity Index, whereas in clinical practice, it is defined as the absence of any gut-related symptoms, with normal inflammatory markers and blood parameters. Mucosal healing can be defined as the absence of deep ulcers, complete absence of ulcers or erosions, or no inflammation.

Management of Crohn's disease depends on the site, extent and activity of disease, and the presence of complications. For this reason Part 2 is divided into chapters in which the location of disease (e.g. oral/upper gastrointestinal disease, small bowel disease, localised ileocaecal CD), behaviour of disease (e.g. stricturing or fistulising disease) and complications of disease (e.g. postoperative recurrence) are discussed.

Most chapters have an algorithm which incorporates evidence derived from clinical trials and cohort data into a format that assists clinical decision-making in the management of patients with Crohn's disease, with a view to achieving best possible patient outcomes. Emphasis has also been placed on multidisciplinary team working with gastroenterologists, surgeons, radiologists, specialist nurses, dieticians and pharmacists to achieve optimal individualised patient management.

References

1. Silverberg MS, Satsangi J, Ahmed T, *et al.* Toward an integrated clinical, molecular and serological classification of inflammatory bowel disease: Report of a Working Party of the 2005 Montreal World Congress of Gastroenterology. *Canadian Journal of Gastroenterology* 2005; 19 Suppl A: 5-36.

Chapter 7

Localised ileocaecal Crohn's disease

Simon Peake MRCP Research Fellow and Specialist Registrar, St Mark's Hospital, London, UK
Gareth Bashir MEd FRCS Surgical Registrar, St Mark's Hospital, London, UK
Ayesha Akbar MRCP PhD Consultant Gastroenterologist, St Mark's Hospital, London, UK
Janindra Warusavitarne BMed PhD FRACS Consultant Colorectal Surgeon, St Mark's Hospital, London, UK

Overview

The ileocaecal region is the most commonly affected site in Crohn's disease (CD). Localised ileocaecal Crohn's disease can be treated both medically and surgically. There have been significant advances in both medical and surgical therapies, improving recovery times and patient outcome. The management of patients with localised ileocaecal Crohn's disease should involve a multidisciplinary team approach, including the patient, gastroenterologists, surgeons, dieticians and specialist nurses.

Introduction

The ileocaecal region is the most commonly affected site in Crohn's disease (CD) with 25-30% of CD patients having disease localised to this area [1].

Medical and surgical therapies for CD have greatly improved with time. Increased evidence on the efficacy of immunomodulator therapies (such as thiopurines and methotrexate) and the development of anti-tumour necrosis factor-alpha (anti-TNF-α) agents (including infliximab, adalimumab and certolizumab) has led to these more potent treatments being used more often and earlier in the course of the disease.

The surgical management of ileocaecal CD has improved with minimally invasive surgery, bowel-sparing techniques and enhanced recovery programs. These new measures have led to shorter recovery periods, lower morbidity and superior long-term results.

The threshold for surgery in localised ileocaecal CD is lower than for disease elsewhere; with some experts still advocating surgery (especially with laparoscopic-assisted resection) in preference to medical therapy for disease in this location, with others recommending surgery if medical therapy is not effective within a short time frame.

Medical management of ileocaecal CD

Traditionally, the medical management of CD is a step-up approach, starting with the least toxic agents and adding in more potent agents as required. However, some clinicians feel that this approach uses low efficacy agents for prolonged periods of time while uncontrolled inflammation continues resulting in tissue damage, and therefore prefer a step-down approach, starting with biological therapy and early introduction of immunomodulator therapies [2]. An alternative approach is a 'rapid step-up' approach particularly in patients at high risk for a disabling disease course.

When considering medical treatments for CD, disease activity is used to guide therapy as well as prognostic factors. Establishing disease activity may pose a problem, especially in CD where symptoms (such as pain and diarrhoea) may be due to causes other than active disease, including bacterial overgrowth, bile salt malabsorption and irritable bowel syndrome.

Hence, objective evidence of disease activity should ideally be obtained prior to starting or changing medical therapy [3]. Disease activity can be determined by laboratory tests, endoscopy and imaging. Risks, benefits and treatment options should be discussed with the patient.

Mildly active ileocaecal CD (CDAI score: 150-219)

A significant proportion of CD patients have a mild disease. In the setting of clinical trials, mild disease has been defined as those with a CDAI score of 150 to 219. In an inception cohort of 843 patients diagnosed with CD between 1990 and 1994 (the ISBEN cohort), only a quarter of patients were treated with immunomodulators and 4% with anti-TNF-α therapy during the first 10 years of follow-up [4].

One option for patients with mild disease would be to refrain from active treatment as a systemic review of clinical trials has revealed that 18% (95% CI, 14-24%) of patients entered remission when on placebo alone [5].

Budesonide (an ethylcellulose-coated steroid released in the ileum) is commonly used to induce remission in mildly active localised ileocaecal Crohn's disease at a dose of 9mg daily. A Cochrane Database Systemic Review has shown this to be superior to placebo (relative risk [RR] 1.96; 95% CI, 1.19-3.23) and mesalazine (RR 1.63; 95% CI, 1.23-2.16) [6]. Studies have shown that budesonide 9mg/day induces remission in 51-60% of patients over 8-10 weeks [7, 8]. Although less effective than prednisolone for induction of remission, it is preferred in mild disease as it is associated with fewer side effects (RR 0.64; 95% CI, 0.54-0.76). This is due to a high first-pass metabolism (90%) resulting in low systemic bioavailability of the drug.

The evidence for mesalazine for inducing remission in mildly active CD is conflicting. Some studies have reported remission rates similar to budesonide (62.1% and 69.5%, respectively) [9]. Previous meta-analysis showed no clinically significant effect of mesalazine in the management of mild to moderately active ileocaecal CD compared to placebo [10]. Further studies using high-dose mesalazine are needed to confirm its efficacy for mildly active CD as it has a favourable side-effect profile but current evidence is poor.

Antibiotics (for example, metronidazole and ciprofloxacin) are not routinely used due to their common side effects which arise as a result of the necessity for long-term therapy, as well as lack of evidence for their usefulness in uncomplicated ileal CD. Small trials and case series looking at nutritional therapy have shown them to be only modestly effective and often poorly tolerated by adults, and therefore their use is limited.

Moderately active ileocaecal CD (CDAI score: 220-450)

For moderately active CD, corticosteroids remain the mainstay of treatment for inducing disease remission. Either prednisolone or budesonide can be used, the former being more effective but also being associated with more side effects [6]. Corticosteroids have been consistently shown to be more efficacious than placebo [11].

Although 48% and 32% of CD patients achieve complete and partial remission with corticosteroid therapy [12], only 29% have endoscopic remission [13]. Hence the early introduction of an immunomodulator (azathioprine, 6-mercaptopurine or methotrexate) or biological therapy is likely to be an effective management strategy as well as minimising the steroid-associated complications. In addition, corticosteroids should be prescribed with concomitant calcium and vitamin D supplements. Patients are selected depending on clinical characteristics, previous response to other medical therapies, phenotype and other comorbidities. Certain patient populations may derive great benefit from the early introduction of biological therapy, including steroid-refractory and steroid-dependant patients [2]. Furthermore, the SONIC study published in 2008 has shown that combination therapy with infliximab and azathioprine is more effective than infliximab alone for achieving and maintaining steroid-free remission in patients at an early stage of disease when immunomodulator-naïve [13].

Severely active ileocaecal CD (CDAI score: >450)

The therapeutic strategy for a patient with severe ileocaecal CD should be a joint decision involving the physician, surgeon and patient.

The usual initial treatment of severely active ileocaecal CD is oral or intravenous corticosteroids depending on disease severity. For some patients who have infrequently relapsing disease, restarting steroids with an immunomodulator therapy may be appropriate treatment. Poor prognostic factors may also help guide the decision in terms of early introduction of immunomodulators and/or anti-TNF-α therapy.

In localised ileocaecal CD, anti-TNF-α therapy is generally reserved for patients not responding to initial therapy and for whom surgery is considered inappropriate. Although there are no data looking specifically at ileocaecal CD, studies have shown that continued use of anti-TNF-α therapy is associated with a substantial reduction (about 30% at 12 months) in surgery and hospitalisation for CD [14]. In addition, some groups of patients who are immunomodulator-naïve may benefit from combination therapy with anti-TNF-α and azathioprine for induction of remission, maintenance of remission for up to 1 year and mucosal healing [14].

Occasionally it is difficult to distinguish between active disease and septic complications. Antibiotics such as ciprofloxacin and metronidazole should be used for patients with fevers or focal tenderness, or in cases where imaging has indicated the presence of an abscess, in order to reduce the possibility of inducing sepsis with corticosteroids.

Surgical management of ileocaecal CD

Surgery is the inevitable outcome for approximately 50% of patients with localised ileocaecal CD in the first 10 years of diagnosis, with a 70-80% lifetime risk of surgery [15].

Both British and American guidelines state that surgery should be offered to those patients who have ileocaecal CD refractory to maximum medical therapy, and those with neoplastic/preneoplastic lesions, obstructing stenoses and suppurative complications [15, 16]. The British Society of Gastroenterology guidelines also state that surgery may be considered as primary therapy in patients with limited ileal or ileocaecal disease [15].

Historically, management of ileocaecal CD has focused on symptom control rather than maintaining remission, and medical therapy has been the mainstay treatment [17]. Surgery was reserved for those patients who presented as an emergency or those who developed the aforementioned complications [15, 17]. These cases inherently carried the higher risk of requiring multiple resections, requiring a defunctioning stoma and the possible development of short bowel syndrome. As a result, gastroenterologists were reluctant to refer cases until all avenues of medical therapy had been exhausted [18]. Surgery for ileocaecal CD has been considered a negative outcome.

The paucity of robust scientific research into the efficacy of medical and surgical therapies in ileocaecal CD has meant that management algorithms and guidelines were mainly based on expert opinion, observational studies and quasi-experimental studies [18].

The advent of laparoscopic colorectal surgery in combination with enhanced recovery programmes has been a major advance leading to better outcomes following gastrointestinal surgery [18-21]. The resultant improvements in reduced postoperative pain, reduced hospital length of stay and faster return to normal activities indicate that surgery is a suitable treatment option to consider early in the course of localised ileocaecal CD.

Open versus laparoscopic surgery

Initial research on the efficacy of surgery in localised ileocaecal CD focused on the difference in outcomes between open and laparoscopic surgery.

In a case-matched series of laparoscopic versus open resection there was a significant reduction in hospital stay (4 vs. 7 days, p=0.0001), time to recovery of full bowel function (2 vs. 5 days, p=0.0001) and overall hospital costs ($9,895 vs. $13,268, p<0.001) in the laparoscopic group [21]. These significant cost savings were also found in a randomised trial of laparoscopic versus open ileocolic resection (∈6,412 versus ∈8,196) [22]. This compares to a 1-year course of infliximab or adalimumab costing ∈17,000 and ∈28,751, respectively [18].

In a systematic review of laparoscopic ileocolic resection, the surgical reintervention rate was between 0% and 8.3% [23]. Indications for reoperation were anastomotic leak, intra-abdominal abscess, necrotising wound infection and small bowel obstruction (nine out of 596 patients, mean complication rate 1.5%). The overall morbidity rate was 15.3% (Figure 1).

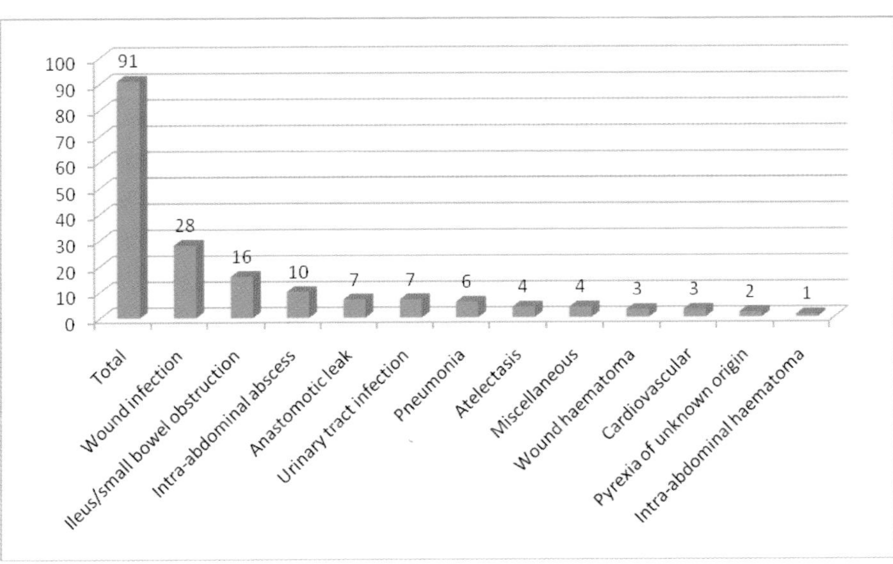

Figure 1. Frequency of in-hospital morbidity in a systematic review of 596 patients undergoing laparoscopic ileocolic resection.

In a national study of 49,609 consecutive ileocolic resections, the in-hospital mortality was significantly better in the laparoscopic group (0.2% vs. 0.9%, $p \leq 0.01$) [24].

Long-term follow-up of a randomised trial of laparoscopic versus open ileocolic resection demonstrated an overall recurrence rate of 52% in 56 patients at a median of 10.5 years [20]. However, only 28.6% required further surgery and only 9% required in-hospital medical treatment. Significantly more patients in the open surgery group required multiple reoperations (12 [44.4%] vs. 3 [10.3%], $p=0.006$) and more patients in the open group required incisional hernia repair although this difference was not significant.

In a further long-term study of laparoscopic-assisted versus open ileocolic resection, the overall recurrence rate in 55 patients at a median follow-up of 6.8 years was 38% and the re-excision rate was 9% [25]. Body image and cosmesis scores were significantly greater in the laparoscopic group.

These two studies demonstrate the long-term efficacy of surgical resection as a treatment for localised ileocaecal CD.

Early versus late surgery

In 1994, 70 patients who had undergone ileocolic resection were questioned regarding their opinion on their surgery. Seventy-four percent of patients answered that they would have preferred their resection to be performed earlier in their clinical course [26]. In a study of open versus laparoscopic ileocolic resection, quality of life in both groups improved significantly at 3 months after resection compared with baseline before surgery ($p<0.0001$) [22].

In a large, multicentre retrospective study of early (surgery at time of diagnosis) versus late (surgery during the course of the disease) ileocolic resection, maintenance therapy with mesalazine was required significantly less frequently in the early surgery group (55% vs. 79%, $p=0.0005$) [27]. There was also a significantly shorter period to disease recurrence and greater frequency of immunomodulator therapy requirement in the late surgery group ($p=0.01$ and $p=0.05$, respectively). Interpretation of this study must be guarded as those in the early surgery group had their

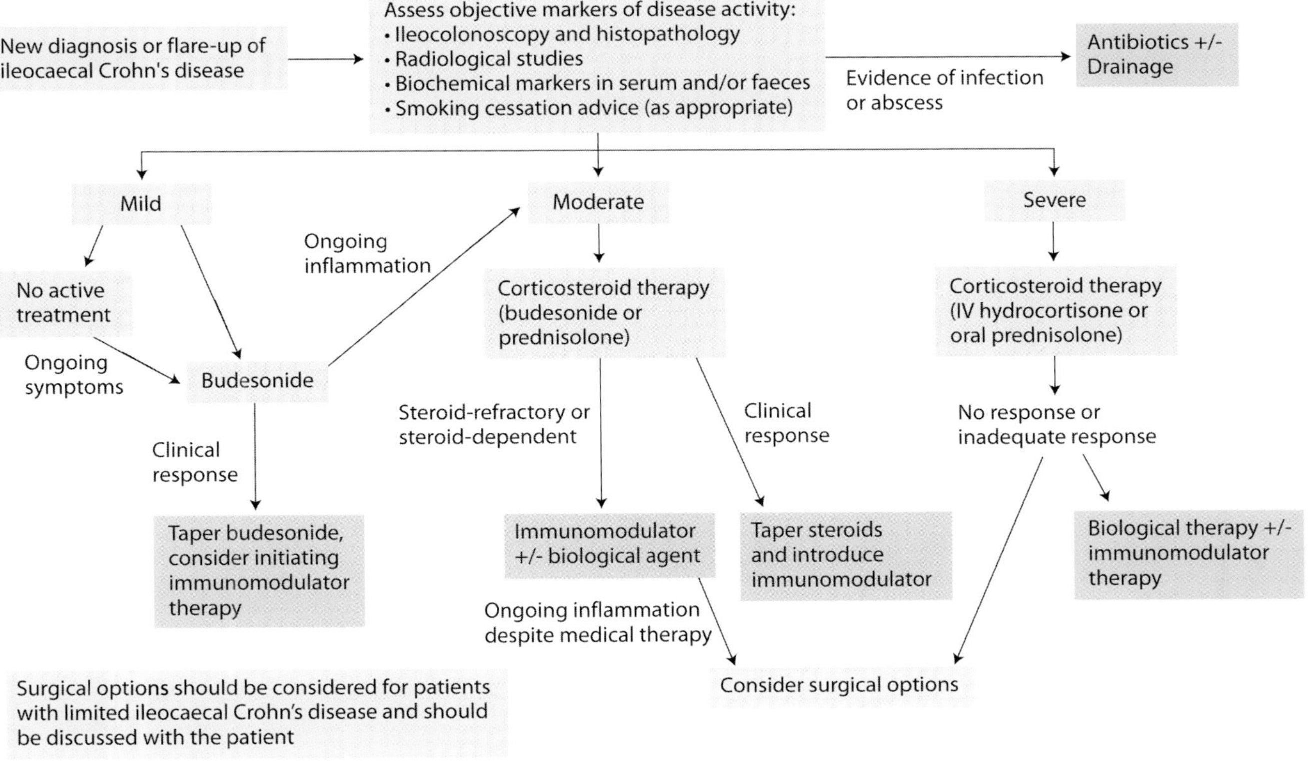

Figure 2. An algorithm for the management of localised ileocaecal Crohn's disease.

resection performed based on clinical need rather than on an assessment of primary treatment and those in the late surgery group had their resection performed based on failed medical therapy.

In 2010, a European consensus paper was published and the guidance relevant to the surgical management of ileocaecal CD is as follows [3]:

- A multidisciplinary approach to the management of CD is recommended and patients should be actively involved in decision-making.
- Surgery should always be considered a treatment option for ileocaecal CD and should be discussed with patients at an early stage.
- Localised ileocaecal CD with obstructive symptoms and no significant evidence of active inflammation should be treated surgically.
- The laparoscopic approach to surgery is the preferred choice where expertise is available.

The long-term efficacy of surgery in localised ileocaecal CD has been demonstrated. Despite this, there is still a lack of research comparing different treatment strategies in terms of efficacy, cost and quality of life (QoL).

The definitive question of who should be offered surgical resection early in the treatment process remains unanswered. However, the outcome of the Laparoscopic Ileocolic Resection Versus Infliximab Treatment of Distal Ileitis in CD trial may provide the answer.

It is clear that current treatment should be individualised for each patient taking into account the patient's QoL, disease activity, treatment efficacy and cost effectiveness. Furthermore, the decision-making process should be multidisciplinary involving the informed patient, gastroenterologist, gastrointestinal surgeon and specialist nurses.

If surgery is to be offered as treatment, extraintestinal manifestations and perianal disease should be excluded as medical therapy is the better option in these circumstances.

An algorithm for the management of localised ileocaecal Crohn's disease is outlined in Figure 2.

Conclusions

The management of localised ileocaecal CD should involve a multidisciplinary approach involving the patient, gastroenterologists, surgeons, dieticians and specialist nurses.

The medical management of localised ileocaecal CD traditionally involves a step-up approach. However, many physicians now favour a step-down approach with the introduction of immunomodulators and biological agents at an earlier stage in the treatment course.

In the era of laparoscopic surgery with enhanced recovery programmes and bowel-sparing techniques, many advocate the role of early surgery in the management of localised ileocaecal CD. Indeed, early surgery is associated with acceptable postoperative morbidity and improved quality of life in the long term.

Key points

- **Management of patients with localised ileocaecal CD should adopt a multidisciplinary approach with treatment decisions involving the patient, gastroenterologist, gastrointestinal surgeon and specialist nurses.**
- **Localised ileocaecal CD can be treated both medically and surgically.**
- **The disease activity and behaviour should be objectively assessed before deciding on the most appropriate medical therapy.**
- **Medical therapy is initiated usually by a step-up approach starting with the least potent agents that will keep disease in remission; however, poor prognostic factors prompt the earlier use of more potent agents or even a step-down strategy.**
- **Surgery in localised ileocaecal CD should be considered as a treatment early in the course of the condition.**
- **Surgery is associated with an acceptable postoperative morbidity rate and disease-free rate at long-term follow-up.**
- **The laparoscopic approach is superior to open surgery.**

References

1. Freeman HJ. Application of the Montreal classification of Crohn's disease to a single clinician database of 1015 patients. *Can J Gastroenterol* 2007; 21: 363-6.
2. D'Haens G, Baert F, van Assche G, *et al.* Early combined immunosuppression or conventional management in patients with newly diagnosed Crohn's disease: an open randomised trial. *Lancet* 2008; 371: 600-67.
3. Dignass A, van Assche G, Lindsay JO, *et al.* The second European evidence-based Consensus on the diagnosis and management of Crohn's disease: current management. *J Crohns Colitis* 2010; 4: 28-62.
4. Froslie KF, Jahnsen J, Mourn BA, *et al.* Mucosal healing in inflammatory bowel disease: results from a Norwegian population-based cohort. *Gastorenterology* 2007; 133: 412-22.
5. Su C, Lichtenstein GR, Krok K, *et al.* A meta-analysis of the placebo rates of remission and response in clinical trials of active Crohn's disease. *Gastroenterology* 2004; 126: 1257-69.
6. Seow CH, Benchimol EI, Griffiths AM, *et al.* Budesonide for induction of remission in Crohn's disease. *Cochrane Database Syst Rev* 2008; 16(3): CD000296.
7. Greenberg GR, Feagan BG, Martin F, *et al.* Oral budesonide for active Crohn's disease. Canadian Inflammatory Bowel Disease Study Group. *New Engl J Med* 1994; 331: 836-41.
8. Thomsen OO, Cortot A, Jewell DP, *et al.* A comparison of budesonide and mesalamine for active Crohn's disease. International Budesonide Mesalamine Study Group. *New Engl J Med* 1998; 339: 370-4.
9. Tromm A, Buganic I, Tomsova E, *et al.* Double-blind, double-dummy, randomised, multicentre study to compare the efficacy and safety of oral budesonide (9mg) and oral mesalazine (4.5g) in moderately active Crohn's disease patients. *Gastroenterology* 2009; 139 (Suppl 1): 391.
10. Hanauer SB, Stromberg U. Oral Pentasa in the treatment of active Crohn's disease: a meta-analysis of double-blind, placebo-controlled trials. *Clin Gastroenterol Hepatol* 2004; 2: 379-88.
11. Benchimol E, Seow CH, Steinhart A, *et al.* Traditional corticosteroids for induction of remission in Crohn's disease. *Cochrane Database Syst Rev* 2008; 2: CD006792.
12. Modigliani R, Mary J-Y, Simon J-F, *et al.* Clinical, biological and endoscopic picture of attacks in Crohn's disease. *Gastroenterology* 1990; 98: 811-8.
13. Colombel JF, Rutgeerts P, Reinisch W, *et al.* SONIC: A randomised, double-blind, controlled trial comparing infliximab and infliximab plus azathioprine to azathioprine in patients with Crohn's disease naïve to immunomodulators and biologic therapy. *J Crohns Colitis* 2009; 3: S45-6.
14. Feagan BG, Pannaccione R, Sandborn WJ, *et al.* Effects of adalimumab therapy on incidence of hospitalisation and surgery in Crohn's disease: results from the CHARM study. *Gastorenterology* 2008; 135: 1493-9.
15. Carter MJ, Lobo AJ, Travis SPL. Guidelines for the management of inflammatory bowel disease in adults. *Gut* 2004; 53 (Suppl V): v1-v16.

16. Lichtenstein GR, Abreu MT, Cohen R, Tremain W. American Gastroenterological Association Institute medical position statement on corticosteroids, immunomodulators, and infliximab in inflammatory disease. *Gastroenterology* 2006; 130: 935-9.
17. Rutgeerts PJ. An historical overview of the treatment of Crohn's disease: why do we need biological therapies? *Rev Gastroenterol* 2004; 4 (Suppl 3): S3-9.
18. Eshuis EJ, Stokkers PCF, Bemelman WA. Decision-making in ileocaecal Crohn's disease management: surgery versus pharmacotherapy. *Expert Rev Gastroenterol Hepatol* 2010; 4: 181-9.
19. Kehlet H, Wilmore DW. Multimodal strategies to improve surgical outcome. *Am J Surg* 2002; 183: 630-41.
20. Stocchi L, Milsom JW, Fazio VW. Long-term outcomes of laparoscopic versus open ileocolic resection for Crohn's disease: follow-up of a prospective randomized trial. *Surgery* 2008; 144: 622-7.
21. Young-Fadok TM, Hall Long K, McConnell EJ, *et al.* Advantages of laparoscopic resection for ileocolic Crohn's disease. *Surg Endosc* 2001; 15: 450-4.
22. Maartense S, Dunkers MS, Slors JF, *et al.* Laparoscopic-assisted versus open ileocolic resection for Crohn's disease: a randomized trial. *Ann Surg* 2006; 243: 143-9.
23. Polle SW, Wind J, Ubbink DT, *et al.* Short-term outcomes after laparoscopic ileocolic resection for Crohn's disease: a systematic review. *Dig Surg* 2006; 23: 346-57.
24. Lesperance K, Martin MJ, Lehmann R, *et al.* National trends and outcomes for the surgical therapy for ileocolonic Crohn's disease: a population-based analysis of laparoscopic vs. open approaches. *J Gastrointest Surg* 2009; 13: 1251-9.
25. Eshuis EJ, Slors JFM, Stokkers PCF, *et al.* Long-term outcomes following laparoscopically assisted versus open ileocolic resection for Crohn's disease. *Br J Surg* 2010; 97: 563-8.
26. Scott NA, Hughes LE. Timing of ileocolonic resection for symptomatic Crohn's disease - the patient's view. *Gut* 1994; 35: 656-7.
27. Aratari A, Papi C, Leandro G, *et al.* Early versus late surgery for ileo-caecal Crohn's disease. *Aliment Pharmacol Ther* 2007; 26: 1303-12.

Chapter 8

Proximal/extensive small bowel Crohn's disease

James Lindsay PhD BM BCh FRCP Senior Lecturer, Barts and the London School of Medicine and Dentistry, Queen Mary University of London; Consultant Gastroenterologist, Barts and the London NHS Trust, London, UK

Part 2

Overview

Proximal gastrointestinal and extensive small bowel Crohn's disease (CD) are more common in patients presenting as children or young adults and often associated with a poor prognosis. All patients require a full history and examination with appropriate investigation to delineate the extent and activity of disease. Few trials focus specifically on proximal or extensive small bowel disease and therefore management plans rely on published guidelines. Early use of immunosuppressive and/or anti-TNF therapy is often required to ensure prolonged mucosal healing and prevent disease progression in this patient group. Nutritional status is a pivotal part of patient assessment and appropriate supplements should be prescribed. Complex patients should be discussed in a multidisciplinary meeting to inform appropriate management plans.

Introduction

The management plan for any patient with Crohn's disease (CD) should take into account the activity, site and behaviour of disease. It is also important to make an assessment of the disease prognosis. It is just as inappropriate to under-treat a patient with poor prognosis disease and risk the complications of disease progression as it is to over-treat a patient with benign disease and put them at risk of drug toxicity. The presence of extensive or stricturing small bowel disease, weight loss at diagnosis and disease onset at a young age are some of the relevant factors that predict the requirement for future surgery, and should be viewed as a mandate for early aggressive therapy. In contrast, mild limited ileal disease that commences in adulthood is often associated with a benign disease course and can often be managed conservatively.

Several management issues are specific to patients with proximal (oral /upper gastrointestinal) or extensive small bowel disease. For example, nutrient deficiencies are common and nutritional therapies form an important adjunct to medical management and may be therapeutic in their own right. Although treatment decisions should be based upon available evidence from clinical trials, there are few data specific to this disease location and therefore appropriate guidelines such as the European Crohn's and Colitis Organisation (ECCO) consensus on the management of CD can be used [1, 2]. In complex cases, the management strategy should be discussed at a multidisciplinary meeting with surgeons, radiologists and allied members of the IBD team. The patient and their family should also be involved in this process wherever possible. This chapter will review the medical and surgical management of both proximal and extensive small bowel disease and discuss an evidence-based therapeutic plan.

Initial investigation

Accurate delineation of the extent and activity of the intestinal involvement in CD is essential to plan appropriate therapy. Investigations should be planned to minimise radiation as patients with extensive disease may require multiple radiological investigations during their disease course and are at high risk of receiving potentially dangerous doses of radiation [3]. It is also important to assess the relevant contribution of fibrosis and inflammation to any intestinal involvement. Thus, although pre-stenotic dilatation suggests an obstructive component, it is essential to correlate the results of investigations with clinical symptoms of obstruction before finalising the management plan. In paediatric practice, the 'Porto agreement' mandates that all newly diagnosed patients undergo complete investigation including upper GI endoscopy, colonoscopy and appropriate small bowel imaging [4]. In adult practice, most patients will undergo colonic and small bowel imaging but upper GI endoscopy is often limited to patients with symptoms that point to disease in the upper GI tract. In addition to endoscopic and radiological imaging, all patients should be assessed for oral involvement. A thorough examination should comment on labial swelling/ulceration, gingivitis, any ulceration of the gums, sulci, palate, tongue and floor of the buccal cavity as well as the presence of deep ulceration and cobblestoning. In addition to routine blood tests to exclude anaemia and assess the inflammatory response, vitamin deficiencies (iron, B12, folate and vitamin D) and coeliac disease should be excluded.

Oral and upper gastrointestinal disease

Reported incidence data for oral and upper GI Crohn's disease vary considerably depending on the definitions used and the population studied. Several cohort studies have suggested that CD in this location is more common in children [5], although this may reflect the increased use of upper GI endoscopy at diagnosis in paediatric practice. Controlled trials of individual therapies in patients with oral and upper GI Crohn's disease are lacking despite the finding that CD in the proximal gut is associated with a worse prognosis. Thus, evidence-based therapy is mainly derived from case series or extrapolated from the management of ileocolonic CD [6].

Medical therapy for oral Crohn's disease

Initial therapy of oral disease revolves around topical therapy with steroids, antibiotics and mild local anaesthetics which can be combined as a mouthwash. More severe cases may require referral to an oral medicine service to consider steroid injections to reduce labial disease. There is limited non-controlled evidence to support the use of topical tacrolimus. An exclusive enteral liquid diet may be beneficial particularly in patients who have co-existent ileocolonic disease, and some centres recommend a cinnamon and benzoate-free diet (extrapolating an open-label dietary intervention study in patients with orofacial granulomatosis [7]). If these measures are ineffective, systemic steroids are used to induce remission with the early introduction of a thiopurine as a steroid-sparing agent. Case reports suggest that anti-TNF agents are effective in the treatment of refractory oral CD [8]. For details on the management of oral CD see Chapter 14.

Medical therapy for upper GI Crohn's disease

Initial therapy for upper GI Crohn's disease revolves around acid suppression with high-dose proton pump inhibitors. It is important to diagnose and eradicate co-existing *Helicobacter* infection. If these measures are ineffective, patients should be commenced on conventional Crohn's therapy with steroids and early introduction of immunosuppressive therapy if a steroid-sparing agent is required. One should have a lower threshold for starting anti-TNF therapy than for disease elsewhere, given the poor prognosis. It is essential to exclude opportunistic infections such as candidiasis and Cytomegalovirus/Herpes simplex virus oesophagitis if upper GI symptoms occur in a patient who is already taking immunosuppressive therapy prior to escalating this treatment.

Extensive small bowel Crohn's disease (Figure 1)

Determining the activity of small bowel disease may be more difficult than for Crohn's colitis, since symptoms (such as pain or diarrhoea) may be due to causes other than active disease. Therefore, alternative explanations for symptoms such as enteric infection, abscess, bacterial overgrowth, bile salt malabsorption, dysmotility (IBS), or gall stones should always be considered. Objective evidence of disease activity should be obtained before commencing or altering medical therapy. As before, the appropriate choice of therapy is influenced by the balance between efficacy and toxicity; previous response to treatment; and the

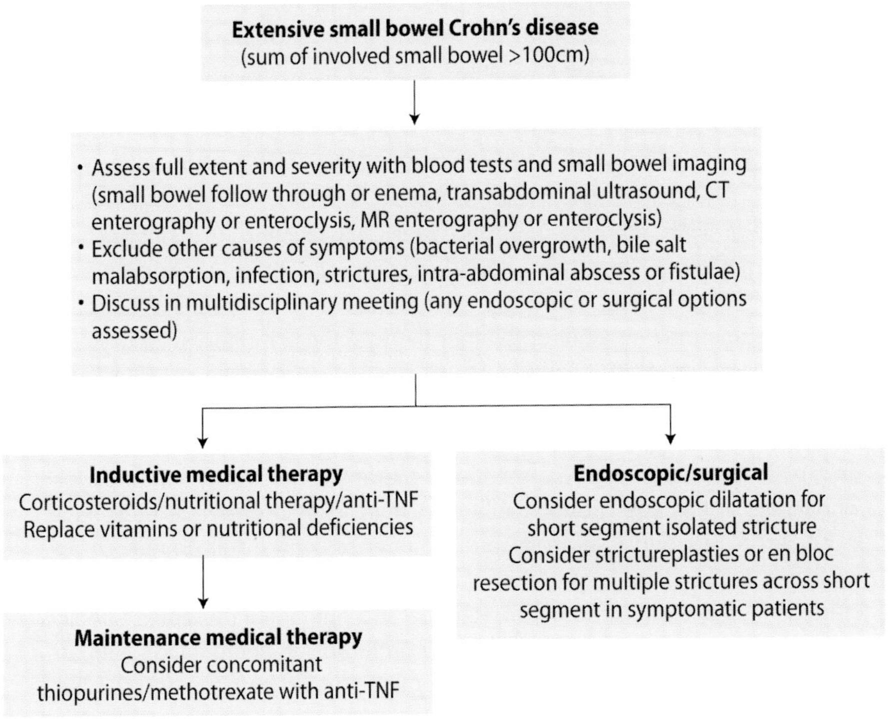

Extensive small bowel Crohn's disease
(sum of involved small bowel >100cm)

↓

- Assess full extent and severity with blood tests and small bowel imaging (small bowel follow through or enema, transabdominal ultrasound, CT enterography or enteroclysis, MR enterography or enteroclysis)
- Exclude other causes of symptoms (bacterial overgrowth, bile salt malabsorption, infection, strictures, intra-abdominal abscess or fistulae)
- Discuss in multidisciplinary meeting (any endoscopic or surgical options assessed)

↓ ↓

Inductive medical therapy
Corticosteroids/nutritional therapy/anti-TNF
Replace vitamins or nutritional deficiencies

↓

Maintenance medical therapy
Consider concomitant
thiopurines/methotrexate with anti-TNF

Endoscopic/surgical
Consider endoscopic dilatation for
short segment isolated stricture
Consider strictureplasties or en bloc
resection for multiple strictures across short
segment in symptomatic patients

Figure 1. Proposed algorithm for the management of extensive small bowel CD.

projected prognosis in the individual patient. The inflammatory burden is greater in extensive (>100cm) than in localised small bowel disease, often resulting in nutritional deficiencies which should be diagnosed and treated.

Increasingly, studies suggest that therapy that allows complete and prolonged resolution of intestinal inflammation reduces the progression to stricturing and penetrating complications, and limit the need for surgery [9]. Therefore, the management plan should incorporate therapies to induce remission and then maintain clinical and mucosal response. Appropriate monitoring to prevent complications relating to drug toxicity and assessing response to therapy is also essential.

Inducing remission in extensive small bowel Crohn's disease

Treatment with steroids and the early introduction of concomitant immunomodulators (for their steroid-sparing effect) is an appropriate therapy although repeat courses should be avoided [1]. Nutritional support may be required as an adjunct to other medical therapy. However, there is clear evidence that an exclusive liquid diet with polymeric or elemental formula feeds can induce clinical remission and reduce the inflammatory activity in patients with ileal CD. In view of the negative impact of steroids on growth velocity in children, nutritional therapy is the first-line therapy for all patients in this age group [2]. Although there is also evidence of benefit in adults, a reduced tolerability and adherence to the full course of an exclusive liquid diet, meant that the published meta-analysis favoured steroids [10]. Patients refractory to steroids and nutritional therapies should be considered for early anti-TNF therapy preferably in combination with an immunosuppressant [11], although surgery should also be considered if the disease is localised.

Maintaining remission in extensive small bowel Crohn's disease

Although it may be appropriate not to use maintenance therapy in some patients with limited small bowel CD, the majority of patients with extensive disease have a poor prognosis and require the early introduction of immunosuppressive therapy with appropriately dosed and monitored thiopurine or methotrexate therapy. Regular review to ensure clinical and mucosal remission is required to tailor therapy and prevent progression to complicated (stricturing/penetrating disease). If patients have ongoing evidence of active disease despite conventional immunosuppressive therapy, escalation to an anti-TNF agent is required once alternative explanations for their symptoms have been excluded. Several analyses have shown that anti-TNF therapy is more effective when treatment is initiated early in the disease. There is clear evidence that combination therapy with an anti-TNF agent and an immunosuppressive such as azathioprine is more effective with both enhanced mucosal healing and reduced immunogenicity in thiopurine-naïve as well as refractory patients [11, 12]. It is likely that multiple immunosuppressive therapies increase infectious complications [13] and may increase the risk of lymphoma. However, it is important to note that the excessive use of steroids is the main driver for infectious complications in many studies [13, 14] and that many of these complications increase with age (particularly in patients over 65 years) [15]. This mandates careful discussion both with an IBD multidisciplinary team and the patient themselves to ensure an appropriate therapeutic plan.

Surgery for extensive small bowel Crohn's disease

The role of surgery for patients with extensive small bowel CD has changed considerably during the last decade as a result of developments in medical therapy and surgical practice (please see ECCO consensus [1]). The evidence on which surgery is based includes very few prospective randomised studies. However, there is good evidence that extensive resection is no longer necessary and potentially harmful due to the risk of nutritional deficiencies relating to short bowel syndrome. Consequently, the current trend is to resect as little as possible even if this results in areas of diseased bowel remaining *in situ*. The rationale for this is that once the part of the bowel responsible for the symptoms has been resected, appropriate medical therapy can be used to control any residual intestinal inflammation. The risk of short bowel syndrome due to extensive bowel resection is thought to be much lower with this strategy. As an alternative to small bowel resection, strictureplasty can be used in jejuno-ileal CD, with similar short-term and long-term results. Most surgeons limit conventional strictureplasties to lengths of intestine <10cm. However, there is increasing experience with novel strictureplasties for diseased areas >10cm that report good results. Where there are multiple strictures in a short segment and where bowel length is sufficient to avoid short bowel syndrome, it may be more appropriate to resect the disease en bloc rather than perform multiple strictureplasties. Intestinal failure due to a structurally short small bowel is more likely to result from multiple operations within a short time span to deal with complications from the primary surgery rather than planned operations over several years for recurrent disease. However, it is important to consider introducing medical therapy with a thiopurine after surgery to prevent disease recurrence. An anti-TNF agent may be considered in selected high-risk patients. Thought should also be given to a scheduled assessment of the anastomosis to exclude significant recurrent inflammation even if the patient is asymptomatic to allow proactive adjustment of medical therapy and prevent the need for recurrent surgery.

When active small bowel CD is associated with an abdominal abscess, percutaneous drainage and delayed resection may be preferable if there are obstructive symptoms. In contrast, drainage followed by medical treatment can be considered if there are no obstructive symptoms. It is important to assess the nutritional status of this group of patients and provide appropriate enteral or parenteral support.

Conclusions

Patients with proximal or extensive small bowel Crohn's disease present significant management challenges in that the disease is often associated with a poor prognosis and there are few appropriately designed clinical trials to aid the formulation of an appropriate therapeutic plan. It is essential to investigate all patients to be clear of the extent of disease, to exclude septic complications and alternative causes for a patient's symptoms, and to delineate the relative contribution of intestinal inflammation and fibrosis to significant strictures. The aim of therapy should be to induce prompt remission and prolonged mucosal healing to prevent progression to complicated disease. Often this will require early introduction of immunosuppressive drugs or anti-TNF therapy. Particular attention should be paid to the nutritional status of the patient and appropriate supplements should be given. Complex patients should be discussed in a multidisciplinary meeting with surgeons, radiologists and allied health professionals to determine optimal care.

Key points

- Proximal and extensive small bowel CD are often associated with a poor prognosis.
- The full extent and severity of disease needs to be clarified with appropriate investigations.
- Nutritional status is a key part of patient assessment and optimising nutrition is important in the management of this group of patients.
- Early use of immunosuppressive and/or anti-TNF therapy is often required in this patient group.
- Patients with complex disease should be discussed in multidisciplinary meetings so that appropriate management plans are formed.

References

1. Dignass A, Van Assche G, Lindsay JO, *et al.* The second European evidence-based Consensus on the diagnosis and management of Crohn's disease: current management. *J Crohns Colitis* 2010; 4: 28-62.
2. Van Assche G, Dignass A, Reinisch W, *et al.* The second European evidence-based Consensus on the diagnosis and management of Crohn's disease: special situations. *J Crohns Colitis* 2010; 4: 63-101.
3. Desmond AN, O'Regan K, Curran C, *et al.* Crohn's disease: factors associated with exposure to high levels of diagnostic radiation. *Gut* 2008; 57: 1524-9.
4. Escher JC, Amil Dias J, Bochenek K, *et al.* Inflammatory bowel disease in children and adolescents. Recommendations for diagnosis: the Porto criteria. Medical position paper: IBD working group of the European Society for Paediatric Gastroenterology, Hepatology and Nutrition (ESPGHAN). *J Pediatr Gastroenterol Nutr* 2005; 41: 1-7.
5. Vernier-Massouille G, Balde M, Salleron J, *et al.* Natural history of pediatric Crohn's disease: a population-based cohort study. *Gastroenterology* 2008; 135: 1038-41.
6. Tremaine WJ. Gastroduodenal Crohn's disease: medical management. *Inflamm Bowel Dis* 2003; 9: 127-8.
7. White A, Nunes C, Escudier M, *et al.* Improvement in orofacial granulomatosis on a cinnamon- and benzoate-free diet. *Inflamm Bowel Dis* 2006; 12: 508-14.
8. Mahadevan U, Sandborn WJ. Infliximab for the treatment of orofacial Crohn's disease. *Inflamm Bowel Dis* 2001; 7: 38-42.

9. Van Assche G, Vermeire S, Rutgeerts P. The potential for disease modification in Crohn's disease. *Nat Rev Gastroenterol Hepatol* 2010; 7: 79-85.
10. Zachos M, Tondeur M, Griffiths AM. Enteral nutritional therapy for inducing remission of Crohn's disease. *Cochrane Database Syst Rev* 2001; 3: CD000542.
11. Colombel JF, Sandborn WJ, Reinisch W, *et al.* Infliximab, azathioprine, or combination therapy for Crohn's disease. *N Engl J Med* 2010; 362(15): 1383-95.
12. Sokol H, Seksik P, Carrat F, *et al.* Usefulness of co-treatment with immunomodulators in patients with inflammatory bowel disease treated with scheduled infliximab maintenance therapy. *Gut* 2010; 59(10): 1363-8.
13. Toruner M, Loftus EV, Harmsen WS, *et al.* Risk factors for opportunistic infections in patients with inflammatory bowel disease. *Gastroenterology* 2008; 134: 929-36.
14. Lichtenstein GR, Feagan BG, Cohen RD, *et al.* Serious infections and mortality in association with therapies for Crohn's disease: TREAT registry. *Clin Gastroenterol Hepatol* 2006; 4: 621-30.
15. Cottone M, Kohn A, Daperno M, *et al.* Advanced age is an independent risk factor for severe infections and mortality in patients given anti-tumor necrosis factor therapy for inflammatory bowel disease. *Clin Gastroenterol Hepatol* 2011; 9: 30-5.

Chapter 9

Colonic Crohn's disease

Paul A. Blaker BSc MBBS MRCP Research Fellow in Gastroenterology, Guy's & St Thomas' Hospital, London, UK
Peter M. Irving MA MD MRCP Consultant Gastroenterologist, Guy's & St Thomas' Hospital, London, UK

Overview

Colonic inflammation occurs in over half of patients with Crohn's disease (CD). Early intervention is necessary since three-quarters of patients with colonic involvement will develop complications within 10 years of disease onset. Accurate assessment of disease activity and extent is the key to tailoring the appropriate therapeutic strategy. 5-aminosalicylic acids and antibiotics are appropriate for mild disease, whereas corticosteroids should be reserved for short-term use in more severe inflammation. Thiopurines and methotrexate can be used as adjunctive treatment in active disease to maintain remission. However, up to one-third of patients are intolerant of, or do not respond to conventional immunosuppressive drugs and alternative interventions including biological agents should be considered. In this chapter we discuss a practical approach to the management of colonic Crohn's disease.

Introduction

Isolated colonic inflammation occurs in 27% of people with Crohn's disease (CD), whereas ileocolonic disease occurs in 24%. Colonic inflammation is usually discontinuous and transmural, commonly with rectal sparing. With disease progression, chronic inflammation leads to irreversible damage, resulting in obstructive episodes, and fistula and abscess formation. After 10 years of disease, penetrating complications are observed in 52% and strictures are found in 20% [1]. Penetrating disease occurs more often (60%) in patients with ileocolonic inflammation.

As with Crohn's affecting any part of the bowel, modern management of Crohn's colitis aims to alleviate symptoms, promote mucosal healing and prolong steroid-free remission, with the aim of altering the natural history of the disease and preventing complications. This should be achieved using interventions of proven efficacy that are appropriate to the severity of the disease and with the best possible side-effect profile.

Diagnosis and assessment

The diagnosis may be suggested by clinical, laboratory and radiographic evaluation but should be confirmed by ileo-colonoscopy. The typical histological findings of granulomas are seen in 51% of patients. In 21%, the inflammation is non-specific and may be difficult to differentiate from ulcerative colitis [2].

Assessing disease severity remains paramount in determining the most appropriate therapeutic strategy. Both the Crohn's Disease Activity Index (CDAI) and the Harvey Bradshaw Index (HBI) have been used to grade disease activity; however, a working definition of severity may be more useful in clinical practice [3] (Table 1).

Plain abdominal X-ray is useful for monitoring fulminant colitis in patients at risk of toxic dilatation but is not a reliable guide of disease extent. Whilst barium enemas may provide more accurate assessment of disease extent, defining stenoses and fistulous tracts not seen on plain X-rays, abdominal

Table 1. Working definitions of Crohn's disease activity [2].
Asymptomatic remission (CDAI <150)
The patient is asymptomatic or without inflammatory sequelae, either spontaneously or after acute medical or surgical intervention
Mild to moderate Crohn's disease (CDAI 150-220)
Ambulatory patients able to tolerate an oral diet without dehydration, toxicity, abdominal pain or tenderness, or weight loss of more than 10%
Moderate to severe Crohn's disease (CDAI 220-450)
Patients failing treatment for mild to moderate Crohn's disease or with prominent symptoms of fever, intermittent nausea or vomiting, abdominal pain or tenderness, significant weight loss or anaemia
Severe fulminant disease (CDAI >450)
Persistent symptoms despite conventional steroid therapy or biological agents as an outpatient, or individuals presenting with high fever, persistent vomiting, intestinal obstruction, signs of peritonism, cachexia, or evidence of an abscess

MRI is emerging as the imaging modality of choice. MRI may differentiate between segments of active and inactive disease and also provides information about extra-luminal structures. Contrast-enhanced high-resolution ultrasound is also effective in imaging active CD and has a role in the initial investigation of Crohn's-related abscesses and inflammatory masses where CT is undesirable. However, in comparison with ultrasound, contrast-enhanced CT scanning provides superior definition of extra-luminal disease and is particularly useful for identifying retroperitoneal complications.

Mucosal assessment is best performed colonoscopically allowing accurate assessment of both the extent and severity of inflammation. The use of validated endoscopic scoring systems (Table 2) may negate the vagaries of colonoscopic evaluation of disease activity and reduce inter-observer bias [4].

Table 2. Simplified endoscopic activity score for Crohn's disease (SES-CD) [4].

	0	1	2	3
Presence and size of ulcers	None	Aphthous <0.5cm	Large 0.5-2cm	>2cm
Extent of ulcerated surface	0%	<10%	10-30%	>30%
Extent of affected surface	0%	<50%	50-75%	>75%
Presence and type of narrowings	None	Single, can be passed	Multiple, can be passed	Cannot be passed

The endoscopic variables are assessed for each of the ileum, right colon, transverse colon, left colon and rectum, and expressed as a total score.

Achieving and maintaining remission

Mild to moderate Crohn's colitis

Smoking

Smoking behaviour is associated with the onset and severity of CD, an increased risk of postoperative recurrence and higher IBD-related mortality. It has been suggested that a higher proportion of non-smokers have colonic disease as compared to current smokers, perhaps suggesting a protective effect of smoking in Crohn's colitis [5]. Notwithstanding this observation, smoking cessation advice should be offered to all patients.

5-aminosalicylates (5-ASAs)

Treatment with 5-ASAs should be reserved for mildly active Crohn's colitis, since they are poorly effective and do not alter the natural history of the disease; treatment with mesalazine (Pentasa 4g/day) results in only a modest reduction in the mean CDAI score (67 points) as compared to placebo [6]. Furthermore, mesalazine does not prevent relapse after corticosteroid-induced remission. In patients with mildly active distal colonic CD, international guidelines suggest the use of topical 5-ASA, although there are little data supporting this [7]. Finally, the role of 5-ASAs in chemoprevention of colorectal cancer remains to be established.

Antibiotics

In patients with mild colitis, treatment with antibiotics is an alternative to 5-ASA. Ciprofloxacin at a dose of 1g per day is equivalent in efficacy to 4g of mesalazine, with complete remission demonstrated in 56% and 55%, respectively [8]. In those treated with metronidazole (10-20mg/kg/day), over half enter clinical remission, whilst uncontrolled data support the use of metronidazole (200-500mg daily) in the maintenance of remission [9]. However, adverse drug reactions, including a disulfram-like effect, peripheral neuropathy and a metallic taste, limit its long-term use.

Budesonide

Budesonide 9mg daily is superior to both placebo and 5-ASA in the management of mildly active proximal colonic inflammation, achieving remission in 51-60% over 8-10 weeks [7]. However, it has no role in the management of distal colonic disease or in the maintenance of remission. Budesonide 9mg/day may be continued for up to 8-16 weeks prior to tapering over 2-4 weeks.

Moderate to severe Crohn's colitis

Conventional therapeutic strategies

Steroids

Systemic corticosteroids are advocated as first-line agents in the management of moderate to severe Crohn's colitis. The National Cooperative Crohn's Disease Study (NCCDS) demonstrated remission rates of 60% at 17 weeks in patients with active CD treated with oral prednisolone (0.5-0.75mg/kg), double that seen in the control group [10]. Furthermore, in 109 patients requiring corticosteroids for acute severe CD, complete remission was achieved in 48%, partial remission in 32% and primary non-response was observed in 20% [11]. Among responders 46% developed a disease relapse and 36% became steroid-dependent within 1 year after commencing treatment.

Following a clinical response to high-dose corticosteroids (prednisolone 40-60mg/day), dosage is usually tapered over several weeks. There is no evidence for any particular withdrawal regimen although many favour a reduction by 5mg per week for simplicity. Adverse events including fluid retention, osteoporosis, adrenal suppression, hyperglycaemia and hypertension, and a failure to maintain remission (probably related to lack of mucosal healing) render maintenance therapy with steroids inappropriate.

Thiopurines

Azathioprine (2-2.5mg/kg) and 6-mercaptopurine (1-1.5mg/kg) demonstrate a corticosteroid-sparing effect in active disease (odds ratio 3.86) [12]. Both therapies are generally well tolerated and promote mucosal healing, maintaining remission in two-thirds of patients. Given the delay in their onset of action (up to 4 months), bridging therapy is usually necessary in active disease. Regular blood monitoring is required to screen for cytopenia and elevation of liver enzymes, which occurs in 1-2% of patients. Thiopurine-S-methyltransferase (TPMT) levels should be checked prior to starting treatment, since low TPMT activity is associated with adverse drug reactions. Monitoring of thioguanine nucleotide (TGN) and methylated thiopurine metabolite levels may allow dose optimisation and predict drug toxicity [13].

Methotrexate

Methotrexate is effective in inducing and maintaining clinical and endoscopic remission. In a controlled study, intramuscular methotrexate, 25mg per week, induced remission in 39% of patients and maintained remission at 40 weeks (15mg per week) in 65%, compared with 19% and 39% given placebo, respectively [14].

Peak onset of methotrexate is typically observed after 12 weeks of treatment. Most series advocate parenteral or subcutaneous methotrexate 25mg weekly (with weekly folic acid 5mg) for 16 weeks, followed by oral methotrexate 15mg weekly. The main adverse effects include bone marrow suppression and hepatotoxicity, therefore monitoring of the full blood count and liver tests are recommended on a 3-monthly basis. In patients with persistently abnormal liver tests, methotrexate should be discontinued and a liver biopsy performed. Methotrexate should be avoided in women of childbearing age being contraindicated in pregnancy.

Biologics

Anti-TNF antibodies (infliximab, adalimumab and certolizumab pegol) are an effective treatment for moderate to severe Crohn's colitis. Remission is achieved in approximately 60% with induction therapy and approximately 50% of patients maintain remission after 1 year of treatment. Anti-TNF drugs result in mucosal healing and, in association with this, a decreased need for hospitalisation and surgery [15]. In patients with a short disease duration, early combined immunosuppression with azathioprine and infliximab appears to be better than standard 'step up' therapy [16]. In addition, at least in thiopurine-naïve patients, combination therapy with azathioprine and infliximab is superior to either drug alone [17].

Treatment with anti-TNF agents appears to be relatively safe. Side effects such as infusion reactions usually respond to slowing the infusion rate or treatment with antihistamines and rarely require corticosteroids. Anaphylactic reactions have been reported but the absolute risk is small. Fortunately, the more worrying side effects such as serious infection, lymphoma and demyelination are rare. Recently, dermatological problems, such as psoriasiform-type rash, have come to light although many of these do not result in discontinuation of treatment.

Severe-fulminant Crohn's colitis

Patients with severe-fulminant colitis require hospitalisation. Treatment with bowel rest, intravenous corticosteroids with or without antibiotics should be commenced. Radiological assessment with ultrasound or contrast-enhanced CT should be performed. Multidisciplinary care with a surgical team is mandatory. In patients with malnutrition or severe fistulising disease, total parenteral nutrition should be considered. Surgery is often necessary.

Alternative therapeutic strategies

A number of other immunomodulatory agents have been advocated in the management of active, refractory colonic CD and are discussed here; however, guidelines for their use have yet to be determined.

Cyclosporine

A systematic review found that standard doses of cyclosporine (5mg/kg/day) did not significantly increase remission rates compared to placebo [18]. Furthermore, there is no evidence to support its role in the maintenance of remission; therefore, the routine use of cyclosporine in colonic CD is not recommended. Uncontrolled data have reported using cyclosporine enemas in resistant proctitis, with low levels of toxicity, which may support its short-term use as a bridge to surgery. Arsenic (acetarsol) suppositories 250mg twice daily for 3-4 weeks may be considered as an alternative to this strategy.

Tacrolimus

A number of uncontrolled small studies have shown that oral tacrolimus is effective in both refractory luminal and perianal fistulising CD [19]. Topical tacrolimus may also have a role in distal colitis. A clinical response may be seen within 2 weeks and therefore it may be used as a bridge to thiopurines. Due to the risk of nephrotoxicity, renal function and serum drug levels should be checked twice-monthly.

Mycophenolate mofetil

Mycophenolate mofetil (MMF) has been advocated in the treatment of thiopurine-resistant patients. However, there is a lack of evidence from controlled trials to support its use. In a UK series of 48 patients with refractory colonic CD, 22% maintained steroid-free remission for a mean duration of 28 months [20]. However, one-fifth of patients stopped treatment due to side effects, including diarrhoea, and at 5 years, over half required additional medical or surgical therapy, suggesting a lack of long-term efficacy. Overall, MMF may have a role in a small number of patients with treatment-refractory disease.

Thalidomide

In treatment-resistant patients receiving a median dose of thalidomide 100mg, 75% of patients with luminal CD demonstrated a clinical response at 12 months [21]. However, half of the patients stopped treatment due to side effects. At present thalidomide is not recommended for the management of colonic CD outside of clinical trials.

Thioguanine

Concerns remain regarding hepatotoxicity and the development of nodular regenerative hyperplasia associated with high-dose thioguanine. However, the use of low-dose thioguanine (20mg) in patients refractory to other immunomodulators is effective and appears to have a better safety profile [22]. MRI or liver biopsy after 12 months of treatment is advised, with regular follow-up to screen for portal hypertension [19].

Anti-mycobacterium paratuberculosis (anti-MAP) therapy

Small open-label studies have suggested that antibiotic therapy against MAP may achieve clinical remission rates. However, whilst a randomised controlled trial of patients with moderate-severe CD treated with a combination of clarithromycin, rifabutin and clofazimine reported an initial benefit after 16 weeks of treatment in comparison with placebo, it was not sustained for up to 2 years [23]. At present, short to medium-term use may be considered in some patients with refractory colitis.

Extracorporeal photopheresis (ECP)

ECP involves the *ex vivo* treatment of apheresed peripheral leukocytes with 8-methoxypsoralen prior to exposure to UVA light, which causes apoptosis. In patients with refractory CD, 12 weeks of ECP results in remission in about half of patients. However, further sham-controlled studies are required before this may be considered a routine intervention.

Trichuris suis therapy

It has been suggested that helminths may protect against and possibly ameliorate CD. In an open-label study including 5/29 and 14/29 patients with isolated colonic and ileocolonic disease, respectively, treatment with *T suis* ova every 3 weeks for 24 weeks, led to disease remission in 72% of patients by week 12 [24]. The treatment is well tolerated and may hold some hope for the future.

Stem cells

In patients with severe refractory CD, phase 1 studies support the use of autologous stem cell transplants and bone marrow-derived mesenchymal stromal cell treatment. Ongoing trials will provide more information regarding the use of stem cell therapy in the near future.

Surgery for colonic Crohn's disease

In some patients surgery may be required to treat complications or induce remission; however, it is not curative. In colonic disease, specific indications for surgery include the formation of strictures leading to partial or complete bowel obstruction, internal fistulae complicated by abdominal abscess, enterovesical fistulae, and enterocutaneous fistulae. Case series have shown that most patients requiring surgery for colonic disease had left-sided disease [25].

In patients with localised colonic disease, limited resection of the affected segment is advised. Whilst this strategy leads to a higher rate of recurrence as compared to proctocolectomy, it may obviate the need for a permanent stoma. In multi-segment colonic disease a subtotal colectomy with an ileorectal anastomosis should be considered. Abscesses may sometimes be treated with intravenous antibiotics and radiological drainage allowing optimisation of the patient prior to surgery. Colonic strictureplasty is not recommended since, in comparison with small bowel strictures, there is an increased risk of cancer. In mild to moderate stenosing disease, endoscopic dilatation and yearly surveillance is acceptable.

Ileal pouch-anal anastomosis has been considered in selected patients requiring a colectomy for Crohn's colitis. However, due to the high rate of complications and pouch failure, end ileostomy formation should remain the standard treatment.

The optimum strategy for maintenance of remission after colonic surgery remains to be established. Metronidazole (20mg/kg/day) demonstrates short-term efficacy and is typically given for 3 months after an ileocolic resection with primary anastomosis. Mesalazine, budesonide and systemic corticosteroids are of no benefit. In patients considered at high risk of disease recurrence, empirical treatment with thiopurines or anti-TNF agents may be considered. Indeed in patients receiving infliximab for 1 year post-ileocolic resection, histological and endoscopic recurrence of Crohn's is significantly attenuated [26].

Conclusions

The management of colonic Crohn's disease usually requires indefinite therapy to maintain remission, with regular monitoring to check for disease progression. Interventions should be appropriate to disease severity. Patients with disease refractory to conventional treatments remain a clinical challenge. Whilst several new therapeutic options are available, few have been studied in controlled trials. The decision to start such treatments should be made on an individual basis between the multidisciplinary team and the patient, after assessing the risks and benefits of treatment and exploring alternative options including surgery.

An algorithm for the management of colonic Crohn's disease is outlined in Figure 1.

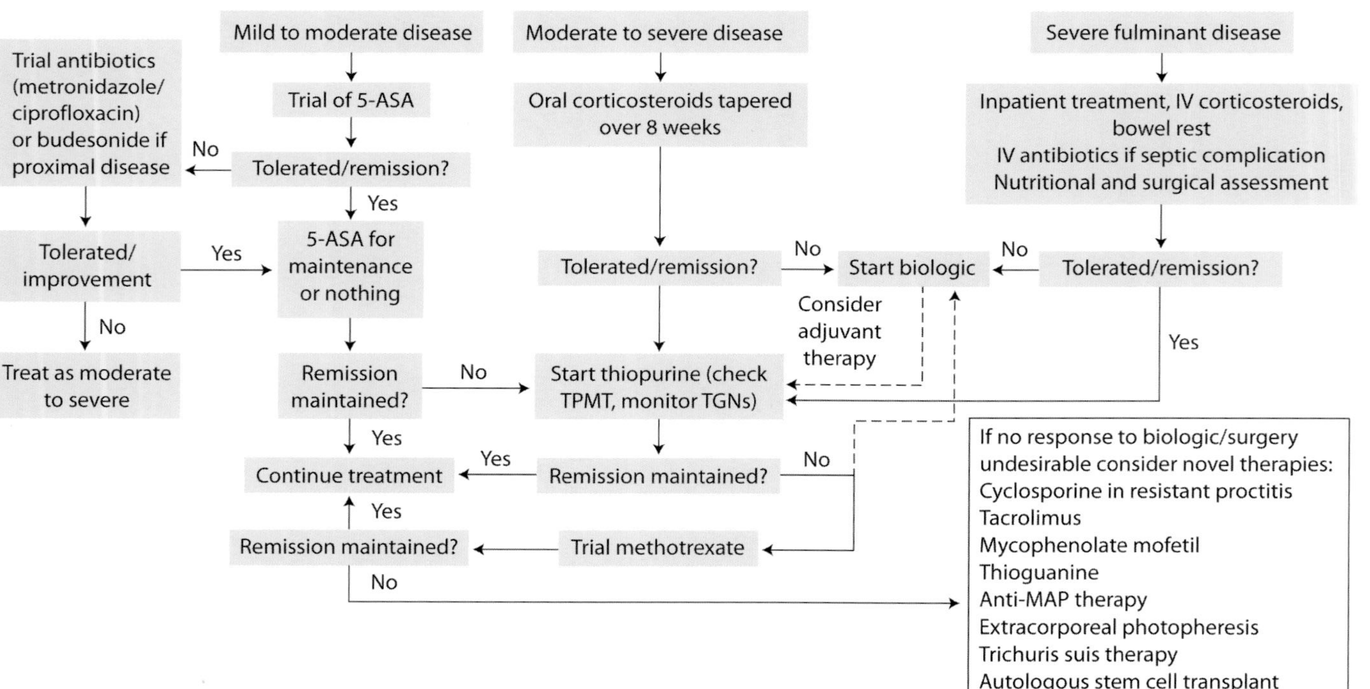

Figure 1. Algorithm for the management of colonic Crohn's disease.

Key points

- A quarter of patients with CD have isolated colonic involvement.
- Accurate endoscopic evaluation of disease activity and extent helps determine the most appropriate therapeutic strategy and allows assessment of mucosal healing.
- Evidenced-based management of colonic CD is complicated by the heterogeneity of CD subtypes included in clinical trials.
- An early 'step-up' in therapy to prevent disease complications should be considered in those failing to respond to initial treatments.
- Surgery is appropriate for disease complications or in those with disease refractory to medical management.

References

1. Louis E, Collard A, Oger AF, *et al.* Behaviour of Crohn's disease according to the Vienna classification: changing pattern over the course of the disease. *Gut* 2001; 49: 777-82.
2. Williams WJ. Histology of Crohn's syndrome. *Gut* 1964; 5: 510-6.
3. Lichtenstein GR, Hanauer SB, Sandborn WJ. Management of Crohn's disease in adults. *Am J Gastroenterol* 2009; 104: 465-83.
4. Daperno M, D'Haens G, Van Assche G, *et al.* Development and validation of a new, simplified endoscopic activity score for Crohn's disease: the SES-CD. *Gastrointest Endosc* 2004; 60: 590-1.
5. Aldhous MC, Drummond HE, Anderson N, *et al.* Does cigarette smoking influence the phenotype of Crohn's disease? Analysis using the Montreal Classification. *Am J Gastroenterology* 2007; 102: 577-88.
6. Hanauer SB, Stromberg U. Oral Pentasa in the treatment of active Crohn's disease: a meta-analysis of double-blind, placebo-controlled trials. *Clin Gastroenterol Hepatol* 2004; 2: 379-88.
7. Travis SPL, Stange EF, Lemann M, *et al.* European evidence-based Consensus on the diagnosis and management of Crohn's disease: current management. *Gut* 2006; 55 Suppl 1: i6-i35.
8. Colombel JF, Lemann M, Bouhnik Y, *et al.* A controlled trial comparing ciprofloxacin with mesalazine for the treatment of active Crohn's disease. *Gastroenterology* 1997; 112: A951 (Abstract).

9. Ursing B, Alm T, Barany F, *et al.* A comparative study of metronidazole and sulfasalazine for active Crohn's disease: the cooperative Crohn's disease study in Sweden. II. Result. *Gastroenterology* 1982; 83: 550-62.
10. Irving PM, Gearry RB, Sparrow MP. Review article: appropriate use of corticosteroids in Crohn's disease. *Alimet Pharmacol Ther* 2007; 26: 313-29.
11. Munkholm P, Langholz E, Davidsen M, *et al.* Frequency of glucocorticoid resistance and dependency in Crohn's disease. *Gut* 1994; 35: 360-2.
12. Sandborn W, Sutherland L, Pearson D, *et al.* Azathioprine or 6-mercaptopurine for inducing remission of Crohn's disease (Cochrane review). In: The Cochrane Library, Issue 1. Oxford, UK: Update Software, 2000.
13. Haines ML, Ajlouni Y, Irving PM, *et al.* Clinical usefulness of therapeutic drug monitoring of thiopurines in patients with inadequately controlled inflammatory bowel disease. *Inflamm Bowel Dis* 2011; 17: 1301-7.
14. Feagan BG, Fedorak RN, Irvine EJ, *et al.* A comparison of methotrexate with placebo for the maintenance of remission in Crohn's disease. North American Crohn's Study Group Investigators. *N Engl J Med* 2000; 342: 1627-32.
15. Schnitzler F, Fidder H, Ferrante M, *et al.* Long-term outcome of treatment with infliximab in 614 patients Crohn's disease patients: results from a single centre cohort. *Gut* 2008; 58: 492-500.
16. D'Haens G, Baert F, Assche G, *et al.* Early combined immunosuppression or conventional management in patients with newly diagnosed Crohn's disease: an open randomised trial. *Lancet* 2008; 371: 660-7.
17. Colombel JF, Sandborn WJ, Reinisch W, *et al.* Infliximab, azathioprine, or combination therapy for Crohn's disease. *N Engl J Med* 2010; 362: 1383-95.
18. McDonald JW, Feagan BG, Jewell D, *et al.* Cyclosporine for induction of remission in Crohn's disease. In: The Cochrane Library, Issue 1. Chichester, UK: John Wiley & Sons, Ltd, 2007.
19. Ng SC, Chan FKL, Sung JJY. Review article: the role of non-biological drugs in refractory inflammatory bowel disease. *Aliment Pharmacol Ther* 2011; 33: 417-27.
20. Ford AC, Towler RJ, Moayyedi P, *et al.* Mycophenolate mofetil in refractory inflammatory bowel disease. *Aliment Pharmacol Ther* 2003; 17: 1365-9.
21. Plamondon S, Ng SC, Kamm MA. Thalidomide in luminal and fistulizing Crohn's disease resistant to standard therapies. *Aliment Pharmacol Ther* 2007; 25: 557-67.
22. Ansari A, Elliott T, Fong F, *et al.* Further experience with the use of 6-thioguanine in patients with Crohn's disease. *Inflamm Bowel Dis* 2008; 14: 1399-405.
23. Selby W, Pavli P, Crotty B, *et al.* Two-year combination therapy with clarithromycin, rifabutin and clofazimine for Crohn's disease. *Gastroenterology* 2007; 132: 2313-9.
24. Summers RW, Elliott DE, Urban JF, *et al. Trichuris suis* therapy in Crohn's disease. *Gut* 2005; 54: 87-90.
25. Tonelli F, Paroli GM. Colorectal Crohn's disease: indications to surgical treatment. *Ann Ital Chir* 2003; 74: 665-72.
26. Regueiro M, Schraut W, Baidoo L, *et al.* Infliximab prevents Crohn's disease recurrence after ileal resection. *Gastroenterology* 2009; 136: 441-50.

Chapter 10

Prevention of postoperative recurrence of Crohn's disease

Lachlan R. O. Ayres MBChB MRCP(UK) Gastroenterology and General (Internal) Medicine Specialty Registrar, Bristol Royal Infirmary, Bristol, UK
Chris S. J. Probert MD FRCP FHEA Professor of Gastroenterology, University of Bristol, School of Clinical Science, Bristol Royal Infirmary, Bristol, UK

Overview

Three-quarters of patients with Crohn's disease (CD) require at least one intestinal resection in their disease course. Even following resection of all macroscopically affected tissue, disease usually recurs at the anastomosis or neo-terminal ileum within weeks to months. Drugs that have been used to prevent recurrence include 5-aminosalicylic acids, nitro-imidazole antibiotics, thiopurines and anti-TNF agents. Optimal management in the postoperative setting involves risk stratification and endoscopic monitoring for recurrence. A further treatment strategy can subsequently be based on these assessments.

Introduction

Disease recurrence after surgery is a great cause of concern amongst patients and clinicians. Many patients require recurrent surgery. The management of Crohn's disease (CD) following surgery requires an individualised approach combined with knowledge of the patterns of disease, risk of recurrence and efficacy of the therapies currently available. The use of preventative treatment creates a dilemma and will expose some patients who may never have required prophylaxis to potentially toxic drugs. However, a policy of watchful waiting will leave some patients under-treated and, with time, results in significant morbidity and complications which could be avoidable. We aim to summarise the evidence for, and to provide a practical approach to, the management of patients with postoperative Crohn's recurrence.

Rate of recurrence

Crohn's disease continues to follow a relapsing-remitting course following intestinal resection. Relapse is most common just proximal to, and at, the anastomosis. The relapse rates are high and there is a plethora of follow-up data to show this [1-4]. The rate of relapse depends on the endpoint used. Endoscopic recurrence occurs more frequently than clinical recurrence and surgical recurrence. At 1 year following ileal resection, 73% of patients had recurrent endoscopic lesions in the neo-terminal ileum, but only 20% had symptoms. At 3 years these figures increased to 85% and 34%, respectively [1].

Repeated surgery in the first few years after resection is the exception rather than the rule. One retrospective study with follow-up data of 139 patients treated with ileocaecal resection showed that repeated surgery occurred in 35% of patients, with a median interval between operations of 7.2 (4.9-10.8) years [2]. Furthermore, 14% of this cohort required two or more resections. In another large series, 46.3% of patients had a second intestinal resection after a median of 5.9 years (71 months) [5].

A meta-analysis of postoperative recurrence in patients receiving placebo in randomised controlled trials for CD was published in 2008 [6].

The pooled estimate of patients experiencing clinical or severe endoscopic recurrence was 24% (95% CI, 13-35; range 0-78). Severe endoscopic recurrence (defined as a Rutgeerts score ≥2) (Table 1) alone was seen in 50% of patients (95% CI, 28-73). Excluding the two outlier studies with the lowest and highest endoscopic recurrence rates, approximately one half of patients developed severe endoscopic recurrence within 3 years (timing of endoscopic assessment ranged from 3-36 months). Even allowing for variability in the follow-up period, there was still a wide range of endoscopic relapse rates (e.g. follow-up at 12 months clinical relapse 10-38%). The differing relapse rates observed are probably due to heterogeneity of the cohorts; in some of the studies there were no data on the site of disease, smoking status or the indication for surgery. Furthermore, the endpoint of endoscopic severity is inevitably subject to a degree of inter-observer variability and scoring systems cannot fully eliminate subjectivity. Finally, only small numbers of patients were included in the studies; the mean number of patients in the placebo arms of the 15 trials included in the meta-analysis was 49. In an unpredictable, relapsing-remitting condition larger numbers of patients are required to reduce the variability encountered.

Table 1. Rutgeerts endoscopic severity score [1].

Grade 0	Normal distal ileum
Grade 1	Up to five small aphthous ulcers
Grade 2	Six or more aphthous lesions with normal mucosa in between or larger lesions with skip areas either at the ileocolonic anastomosis or proximal to it
Grade 3	Diffuse aphthous ileitis with diffusely inflamed mucosa
Grade 4	Diffuse inflammation with larger ulcers, nodules and/or narrowing

Risk factors for recurrence postoperatively

Current cigarette smokers are at high risk of recurrent disease postoperatively (or after remission has been achieved medically) [7]. In a postoperative cohort of 174 patients, Sutherland *et al* demonstrated a 5- and 10-year surgical recurrence rate of 36% and 70%, respectively, for smokers versus 20% and 41% for non-smokers [7]. This effect appears to be more pronounced in females (OR 4.2) than males (OR 1.5). In another case series, smoking was found to be an independent predictor of clinical recurrence (hazard ratio 1.46) and surgical recurrence (hazard ratio 2.0) [8].

Patients with a history of colonic and small bowel involvement [3, 9] and those with penetrating/perforating disease are also at increased risk [4]. Isolated small bowel disease appears to carry the lowest risk.

A meta-analysis suggests that the presence of granulomas is associated with a modestly increased risk of recurrence, repeated surgery and a shorter time to recurrence [10]. However, further larger prospective studies are required to confirm this finding.

The clinical course can be predicted by the severity of endoscopic lesions (see Table 1) 1 year after ileal resection; 80% (28/35) of patients with grade 0-1 lesions had no progression at 3 years, and rarely developed symptoms, compared with 92% (28/35) of patients with grade 3-4 lesions who had a stable or higher endoscopic score at 3 years and were more likely to develop early symptoms, complications and require a second operation [1].

Other factors which have previously been associated with a high risk for recurrent disease but are not fully supported by the available evidence are age, gender, duration of disease, history of surgical resection and resection margins of affected bowel.

Finally, some patients may not be considered high risk in terms of the above risk factors, but a low threshold for treatment may be justified if there is a history of extensive intestinal resection and for whom further surgery would render them with a short bowel and prone to malabsorption.

Monitoring for recurrence

Given the lag time of months to years between the development of endoscopic lesions and clinical symptoms, we recommend that imaging of the small bowel (with ileocolonoscopy or small bowel MRI) should be considered at 6 months after surgery to assess for recurrence and the severity of recurrence which helps to determine further medical management. The ECCO (European Crohn's and Colitis Organisation) guidelines suggest that ileocolonoscopy should be performed if it will alter management [11].

In the presence of symptoms postoperatively, the patient should be fully assessed to determine the cause of the symptoms. Postoperatively there are alternative explanations for the development of symptoms which do not necessarily indicate active disease/recurrence, e.g. adhesions, fibrotic stricture, bile salt malabsorption, irritable bowel syndrome, enteric infections and *Clostridium difficile* infection. Non-invasive methods such as blood testing for inflammatory markers can be supplemented with faecal calprotectin or lactoferrin. Stool cultures can assess for enteric infections. Bile salt malabsorption can be assessed using a SeHCAT scan (selenium homocholic acid taurine). Small bowel imaging can provide further evidence of the underlying disease process (inflammatory disease, fibrotic stricture, adhesions). The gold standard test is ileocolonoscopy.

Drugs

Medical therapy is used to prevent recurrence, induce remission and maintain remission.

5-aminosalicylates (5-ASAs)

A Cochrane review [12] concluded that 5-ASAs are not effective for the maintenance of medically-induced remission. A meta-analysis in 2002 suggests that 5-ASAs reduce the rate of endoscopic recurrence by 18% (NNT=5.5) and clinical recurrence by 15% (NNT=6.6) [13]. The largest study (n=318) examining 5-ASAs for postoperative Crohn's prophylaxis did not find any difference in relapse rates at 18 months comparing 5-ASA (Pentasa) 4g/day versus placebo. A retrospective analysis of patients with isolated small bowel disease showed a significant reduction in clinical recurrence in patients treated with mesalazine compared with placebo (22% versus 40%) [14]. A randomised controlled trial failed to show any significant difference in clinical recurrence at 12 months between 2.4g and 4g of mesalazine (Asacol) daily [15]. More recently in 2009, a Cochrane review on post-surgical recurrence using some of the above data and a later study showed that mesalazine therapy significantly reduced clinical and severe endoscopic recurrence, generating a NNT=12 and a NNT=8 for clinical and severe endoscopic recurrence, respectively [16].

At present, there is only modest evidence to support the routine use of 5-ASAs in the prevention of postoperative recurrence. Inconsistencies between studies have been compounded by the use of different 5-ASA preparations with different release mechanisms, differences in dosages, and duration of follow-up.

Antibiotics

Antimicrobials may be used as an adjunct or alone to prevent disease recurrence. A double-blind controlled study showed that 3 months of oral metronidazole (20mg/kg/day) started 1 week after intestinal resection reduced the risk of severe endoscopic recurrence (13% versus 43%) and clinical recurrence (4% versus 25%) compared with placebo at 1 year [17]. This effect was not sustained at 2 or 3 years. Ornidazole was more effective than placebo in reducing clinical recurrence at 1 year, but results were not different at 3 years [18]. A recent study showed that 3 months of metronidazole together with azathioprine was superior to metronidazole alone in reducing endoscopic recurrence at 12 months in patients at high risk of recurrence [19]. A Cochrane review in 2009 showed that nitroimidazole antibiotics appear to reduce risk of clinical and endoscopic recurrence when compared with placebo with a NNT=4 for both clinical and endoscopic recurrence [16]. The risk of neuropathy limits the use of metronidazole to short periods in clinical practice and, overall, nitroimidazole antibiotics are associated with a high risk of adverse events.

Thiopurines

Three controlled studies have evaluated the role of azathioprine or 6-mercaptopurine in the postoperative setting with variable results [20-22]. Recent retrospective data from 326 patients showed that the group receiving azathioprine had a hazard ratio of 0.41 for surgical recurrence (most patients were observed for 4-5 years) [5]. The greatest risk reduction occurred in patients treated with thiopurines for ≥36 months as compared to 3-35 months or no thiopurines.

Meta-analysis of four controlled trials assessing thiopurines (azathioprine n=3, mercaptopurine n=1) in postoperative CD was published in 2009 [23]. At 1 year, clinical recurrence was reduced in the thiopurine treatment arm compared with the control arm, with a mean difference of 8%, giving a NNT=13. Withdrawal rates were significantly higher in the thiopurine treatment groups than control groups: 17.2% versus 9.8%. Surgical recurrence was not evaluated.

In a recent head-to-head comparison of azathioprine versus mesalazine (4g/day) in patients with moderate to severe endoscopic recurrence 6-24 months after resection and ileocolonic anastomosis [24], none of the patients treated with azathioprine (n=41) developed symptoms compared with 11% (4/37) of patients treated with mesalazine. Adverse drug reactions occurred more frequently in the azathioprine group leading to drug discontinuation in 22%. There was no placebo control in this group of patients who were at high risk of clinical recurrence and the follow-up was relatively short (1 year). Due to drug discontinuation, overall superiority of azathioprine could not be demonstrated; however down-staging of the Rutgeerts score occurred more frequently with azathioprine (19/30, 63%) than mesalazine (11/32, 34%). A Cochrane review in 2009 showed that thiopurines significantly reduced the risk of clinical and endoscopic recurrence compared with placebo, with a NNT of 7 and 4 for clinical and endoscopic recurrence, respectively [16]. Overall, there have been mixed results in the studies of thiopurines and some studies have, on reflection, used an inadequate dosing regime and there are significant drop-out rates due to side effects.

Probiotics

Four placebo-controlled trials have assessed the use of probiotics or synbiotics in the prevention of CD postoperative recurrence.

Two studies showed that daily treatment with *Lactobacillus johnsonii* (LA1) had no benefit in preventing endoscopic recurrence at 3-6 months after ileocaecal resection [25, 26]. *Lactobacillis* GG [27] and synbiotic 2000 [28] were not effective in the prevention of endoscopic recurrence at 12 months.

Overall, there is insufficient evidence to advocate use of probiotics in the prevention of postoperative recurrence of CD.

Anti-TNF drugs

To date few studies have evaulated the role of biologics in the post-surgical prophylaxis setting. Regueiro *et al* randomised 24 patients following ileocolonic resection to infliximab (5mg/kg) or placebo 4 weeks after surgery. Treatment was continued for 1 year at which stage patients were assessed for clinical and endoscopic recurrence. There was no significant decrease in clinical recurrence; however, endoscopic recurrence was significantly reduced: 1/11 in the infliximab group versus 11/13 in the placebo group. Histological recurrence was also significantly lower in the infliximab group: 3/11 versus 11/13 in the placebo group. There were no increased adverse events in this short follow-up period [29]. In the following 12 months, 7/13 patients who had received placebo initially received infliximab and 71% were in remission at 2-year follow-up [30].

In a prospective long-term cohort study, 12 consecutive patients with CD who were treated with maintenance infliximab 5mg/kg immediately after surgery and who had no clinical or endoscopic disease recurrence after 24 months were followed up for an additional 1 year. Infliximab treatment was then discontinued. None of the patients had clinical or endoscopic recurrence 3 years after surgery, but 83% developed endoscopic recurrence when infliximab was discontinued. These data suggest that long-term maintenance therapy may be required to maintain mucosal integrity following surgery [31].

Smoking cessation

In addition to the medical therapies mentioned above, patients with CD should be strongly advised to stop smoking. Many patients are unsuccessful at giving up smoking. Patients may benefit from assistance from their GP, enrolment in smoking cessation groups and the use of medical therapies to aid smoking cessation. Although this has significant resource implications, we speculate it is likely to be cost effective in the long term and will have additional health benefits.

Ongoing/future studies

In view of inconsistent results from previous trials investigating the efficacy of thiopurines, the TOPPIC trial [32] (Trial of Prevention of Post-Operative Crohn's Disease) is a multicentre, randomised controlled trial aiming to recruit 234 patients in the UK. Patients will be treated with 6-mercaptopurine (6MP) 1.5mg/kg or placebo. Patients will be followed up for 3 years and assessed for clinical and endoscopic recurrence. The investigators also aim to shed light on some other interesting clinical questions, such as the effectiveness of faecal calprotectin for diagnosing recurrence, and analysing genetic markers to attempt to identify a high-risk genotype.

Although results of anti-TNF agents in the postoperative setting appear promising, the use of anti-TNF drugs routinely to prevent recurrence in all patients after ileocaecal resection is likely to result in over-treatment of some patients who are at low risk of recurrence. Future studies should assess the use of anti-TNF agents in selected high-risk patients, including those who have failed an immunosuppressive drug.

Conclusions

Management must be individualised depending on the patient's risk factors. Smoking is the only modifiable risk factor and patients should be strongly encouraged to stop smoking. Symptoms of active disease should be correlated with objective evidence of recurrent disease. Patients with severe endoscopic recurrence are likely to run a more aggressive course. There is limited evidence for the use of thiopurines in preventing postoperative recurrence, and further – adequately powered – studies are in progress. If used, thiopurines should be given at an adequate dose for at least 3 years. Evidence for 5-ASA drugs in preventing postoperative recurrence is conflicting and the evidence for a role in isolated small bowel disease is limited. Probiotics are not effective and antibiotics are not a long-term option in view of the side effects and the inability of patients to tolerate the drugs. In high-risk patients where thiopurines are contraindicated or have previously been ineffective or caused intolerable side effects, there are small studies to support the use of infliximab.

Proposed treatment algorithm

In an unpredictable heterogeneous condition, treatment decisions rely in part on judgment and experience. However, a useful strategy for the postoperative Crohn's patient is shown in Figure 1.

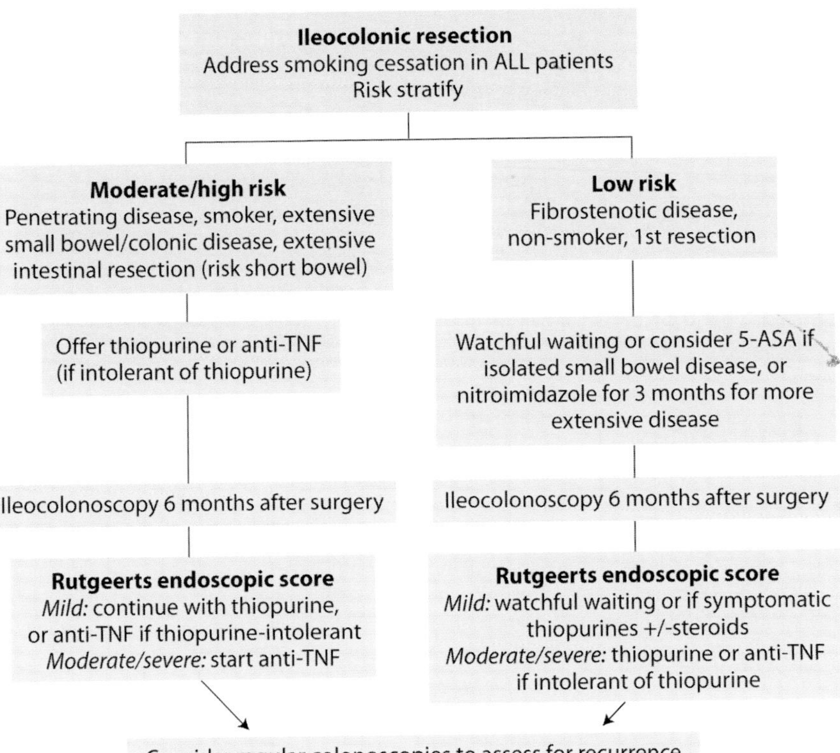

Figure 1. Proposed algorithm to risk stratify patients and to monitor for recurrence.

Key points

- **Risk stratification is important to individualise management of patients with CD in the postoperative setting. Disease location prior to surgery, disease behaviour and smoking are predictive risk factors for recurrence post-surgery.**
- **Endoscopic assessment with ileocolonoscopy is advocated for assessing recurrence.**
- **Antibiotics prevent early endoscopic recurrence and delay clinical recurrence but are often poorly tolerated.**
- **Thiopurines, anti-TNF and 5-ASA drugs can be considered according to the individual patient's risk factors.**

References

1. Rutgeerts P, Geboes K, Vantrappen G, *et al.* Predictability of the postoperative course of Crohn's disease. *Gastroenterology* 1990; 99: 956-63.
2. Cullen G, O'Toole A, Keegan D. Long-term clinical results of ileocaecal resection for Crohn's disease. *Inflamm Bowel Dis* 2007;13: 1369-73.
3. Pascua M, Su C, Lewis J. Meta-analysis: factors predicting postoperative recurrence with placebo therapy in patients with Crohn's disease. *Aliment Pharmacol Ther* 2008; 28: 545-56.
4. Simillis C, Yamamoto T, Reese GE, *et al.* A meta-analysis comparing incidence of recurrence and indication for reoperation after surgery for perforating versus nonperforating Crohn's disease. *Am J Gastroenterol* 2008; 103: 196-205.
5. Papay P, Reinisch W, Ho E, *et al.* The impact of thiopurines on the risk of surgical recurrence in patients with Crohn's disease after first intestinal surgery. *Am J Gastroenterol* 2010; 105: 1158-64.
6. Renna S, Camma C, Modesto I, *et al.* Meta-analysis of the placebo rates of clinical relapse and severe endoscopic recurrence in postoperative Crohn's disease. *Gastroenterology* 2008; 135: 1500-9.
7. Sutherland L, Ramcharan S, Bryant H, *et al.* Effect of cigarette smoking on recurrence of Crohn's disease. *Gastroenterology* 1990; 98(5 Pt 1): 1123-8.
8. Cottone M, Rosselli M, Orlando A. Smoking habits and recurrence in Crohn's disease. *Gastroenterology* 1994; 106: 643-8.
9. Michelassi F, Balestracci T, Chappell R, Block GE. Primary and recurrent Crohn's disease. Experience with 1379 patients. *Ann Surg* 1991; 214: 230-8.

10. Simillis C, Jacovides M, Reese GE, *et al.* Meta-analysis of the role of granulomas in the recurrence of Crohn's disease. *Dis Colon Rectum* 2010; 53: 177-85.
11. Van Assche G, Dignass A, Reinisch W. The second European evidence-based Consensus on the diagnosis and management of Crohn's disease: special situations. *J Crohns Colitis* 2010; 4: 63-101.
12. Akobeng AK, Gardener E. Oral 5-aminosalicylic acid for maintenance of medically-induced remission in Crohn's disease. *Cochrane Database Syst Rev* 2005; 1: CD003715.
13. Camma C, Viscido A, Latella G, *et al.* Mesalazine in the prevention of clinical and endoscopic postoperative recurrence of Crohn's disease: a meta-analysis. *Digestive and Liver Disease* 2002; 34: A86 37 P.
14. Lochs H, Mayer M, Fleig WE, *et al.* Prophylaxis of postoperative relapse in Crohn's disease with mesalamine: European Cooperative Crohn's Disease Study VI. *Gastroenterology* 2000; 118: 264-73.
15. Caprilli R, Cottone M, Tonelli F, *et al.* Two mesalazine regimens in the prevention of the post-operative recurrence of Crohn's disease: a pragmatic, double-blind, randomized controlled trial. *Aliment Pharmacol Ther* 2003; 17: 517-23.
16. Doherty G, Bennett G, Patil S, *et al.* Interventions for prevention of post-operative recurrence of Crohn's disease. *Cochrane Database Syst Rev* 2009; 4: CD006873.
17. Rutgeerts P, Hiele M, Geboes K. Controlled trial of metronidazole treatment for prevention of Crohn's recurrence after ileal resection. *Gastroenterology* 1995; 108: 1617-21.
18. Rutgeerts P, Van Assche G, Vermeire S, *et al.* Ornidazole for prophylaxis of postoperative Crohn's disease recurrence: a randomized, double-blind, placebo-controlled trial. *Gastroenterology* 2005; 128: 856-61.
19. D'Haens GR, Vermeire S, Van Assche G, *et al.* Therapy of metronidazole with azathioprine to prevent postoperative recurrence of Crohn's disease: a controlled randomized trial. *Gastroenterology* 2008; 135: 1123-9.
20. Ardizzone S, Maconi G, Sampietro GM, *et al.* Azathioprine and mesalamine for prevention of relapse after conservative surgery for Crohn's disease. *Gastroenterology* 2004; 127: 730-40.
21. Hanauer SB, Korelitz BI, Rutgeerts P, *et al.* Postoperative maintenance of Crohn's disease remission with 6-mercaptopurine, mesalamine, or placebo: a 2-year trial. *Gastroenterology* 2004; 127: 723-9.
22. D'Haens G, Noman M, Van Assche, *et al.* Severe postoperative recurrence of Crohn's disease is significantly reduced with combination therapy metronidazole + azathioprine: a double-blind controlled randomised trial. *J Crohns Colitis* 2007; 1: 4.
23. Peyrin-Biroulet L, Deltenre P, Ardizzone S. Azathioprine and 6-mercaptopurine for the prevention of postoperative recurrence in Crohn's disease: a meta-analysis. *Am J Gastroenterol* 2009; 104: 2089-96.
24. Reinisch W, Angelberger S, Petritsch W. Azathioprine versus mesalazine for prevention of postoperative clinical recurrence in patients with Crohn's disease with endoscopic recurrence: efficacy and safety of a randomized, double-blind, double-dummy, multi-centre trial. *Gut* 2010; 59: 752-9.

25. Van Gossum A, Dewit O, Louis E, *et al.* Multicentre randomized-controlled clinical trial of probiotic (*Lactobacillus johnsonii*, LA1) on early endoscopic recurrence of Crohn's disease after ileo-caecal resection. *Inflamm Bowel Dis* 2007; 13: 135-42.
26. Marteau P, Lémann M, Seksik P, *et al.* Ineffectiveness of *Lactobacillus johnsonii* LA1 for prophylaxis of postoperative recurrence in Crohn's disease: a randomised, double blind, placebo controlled GETAID trial. *Gut* 2006; 55: 842-7.
27. Prantera C, Scribano ML, Falasco G, *et al.* Ineffectiveness of probiotics in preventing recurrence after curative resection for Crohn's disease: a randomised controlled trial with *Lactobacillus* GG. *Gut* 2002; 51: 405-9.
28. Chermesh I, Tamir A, Reshef R, *et al.* Failure of Synbiotic 2000 to prevent postoperative recurrence of Crohn's disease. *Dig Dis Sci* 2007; 52: 385-9.
29. Regueiro M, Schraut W, Baidoo L, *et al.* Infliximab prevents Crohn's disease recurrence after ileal resection. *Gastroenterology* 2009; 136: 441-50.
30. Regueiro M, Schraut WH, Baidoo L, *et al.* Two-year follow-up of patients enrolled in the randomized controlled trial (RCT) of infliximab (IFX) for prevention of recurrent Crohn's disease (CD) [abstract]. *Gastroenterology* 2009; 136(Suppl 1): A-522.
31. Sorrentino D, Paviotti A, Terrosu G, *et al.* Low-dose maintenance therapy with infliximab prevents postsurgical recurrence of Crohn's disease. *Clin Gastroenterol Hepatol* 2010; 8: 591-9.
32. Edinburgh Clinical Trials Unit. 2010. TOPPIC. Edinburgh: University of Edinburgh. Available from: http://www.clinicaltrials.ed.ac.uk/trials/toppic/default.asp. Accessed 15/11/10.

Chapter 11

Stricturing Crohn's disease

Edward J. Despott MD MRCP(UK) Advanced Endoscopy Research Fellow, Wolfson Unit for Endoscopy, St Mark's Hospital and Academic Institute, Imperial College London, UK

Janindra Warusavitarne BMed PhD FRACS Consultant Colorectal Surgeon, St Mark's Hospital, London, UK

Chris Fraser MB ChB MD FRCP Consultant Gastroenterologist and Specialist Endoscopist, Wolfson Unit for Endoscopy, St Mark's Hospital and Academic Institute; Honorary Senior Lecturer, Imperial College London, UK

Overview

The transmural inflammation that characterises Crohn's disease (CD) frequently leads to the formation of strictures. The risk of developing this complication has been shown to worsen over time. Despite recent advances in medical management, strictures often develop a fibrotic component that is refractory to medical therapy resulting in the need for endoscopic or surgical intervention. This chapter highlights the natural history of stricturing CD and provides an outline of the currently available medical, endoscopic and surgical options for the management of this common yet challenging clinical condition.

Introduction

Stricture formation in Crohn's disease (CD) constitutes a major part of the disease burden and is a leading indication for surgical intervention and hospitalisation for patients with this condition [1]. The distal small bowel (SB) and ileocolic anastomosis are the most common sites of involvement while colonic stricturing may occur in up to 17% of patients and proximal SB and upper gastrointestinal strictures occur in up to 5% [2]. Although it is unclear why some patients develop stricturing disease while others are spared this complication, several factors such as the severity of CD, its duration, ileal involvement and the presence of NOD2/CARD15 or TNF-SF15 genetic polymorphisms appear to be linked with an increased risk of stricture development [3-5]. There is also a tendency for the CD phenotype to worsen over time; one large series showed that up to 27% of patients progressed from a non-stricturing/non-penetrating phenotype to stricturing disease over a period of 10 years [6]. Despite recent advances in the medical management of CD, stricturing disease remains a challenging issue since most strictures eventually develop a significant fibrostenotic component that is refractory to medical therapy and requires endoscopic or more invasive surgical intervention.

Diagnostic approach

Stricturing disease causes gradual narrowing of the intestinal lumen that may remain clinically silent but often manifests itself sub-acutely with post-prandial bloating, colicky abdominal pain or with the signs and symptoms of frank, acute intestinal obstruction (frequently precipitated by a fibre-rich meal). Three types of CD-related strictures are described: inflammatory, fibrostenotic and anastomotic [7]. The inflammatory and fibrostenotic types illustrate the natural history of CD itself and represent the two ends of a progressive continuum; often there is co-existence of inflammation and fibrosis within the same CD stricture. Although an attempt at quantification of the inflammatory and fibrotic components can prove to be a challenging task, every effort should be made to rule out active inflammation, as this has the potential to respond (at least in part) to medical therapy. Post-surgical anastomotic strictures are often very short, frequently occur in the absence of CD recurrence and tend to be more amenable to endoscopic dilatation [8]. Pointers to active disease may be sought from C-reactive protein (CRP) levels, diagnostic imaging and endoscopic evaluation. While CRP is usually raised in active CD, a rise in its level may be caused by inflammation elsewhere and corroboration with other investigations is advised; also, the CRP level may be normal in the face of active disease in up to 10% of patients [9]. Radiological investigations (Figure 1) that may demonstrate disease activity include

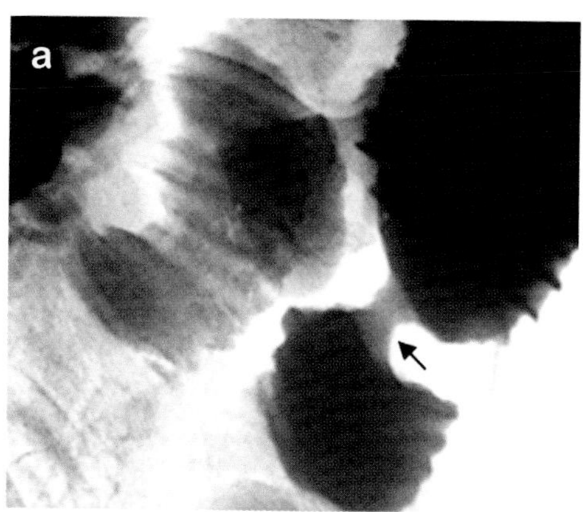

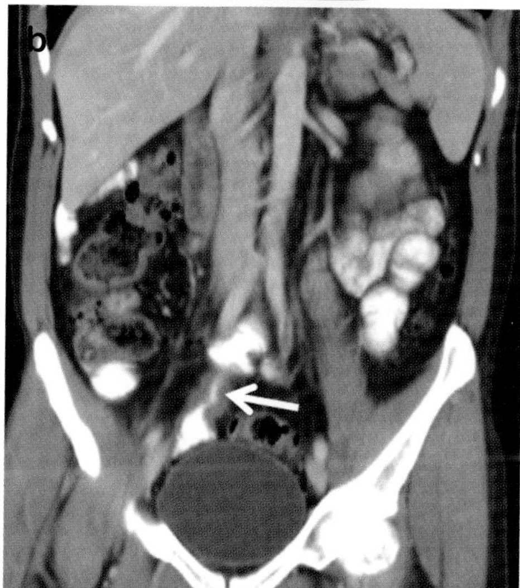

Figure 1. a) Short fibrotic CD stricture as seen at barium follow though and b) computed tomographic enterography. (Different patients.)

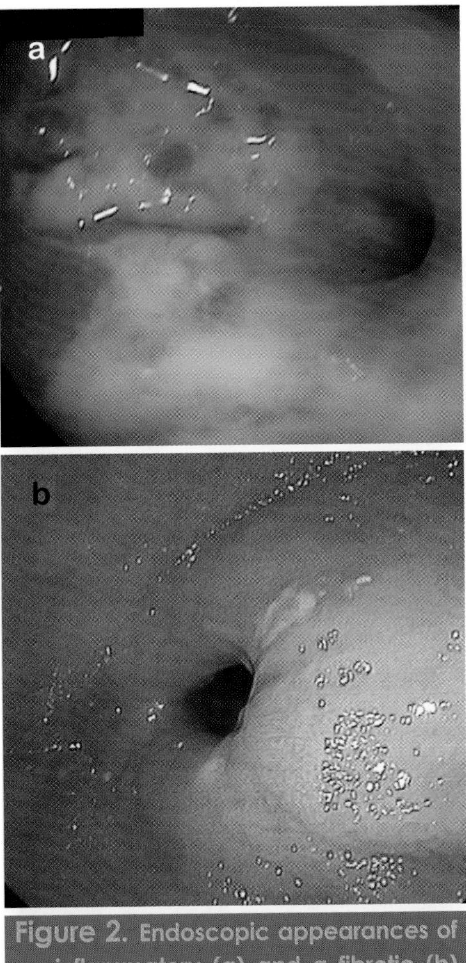

Figure 2. Endoscopic appearances of an inflammatory (a) and a fibrotic (b) CD stricture of the mid-ileum as seen at double-balloon enteroscopy.

barium studies and contrast-enhanced computed tomographic (CT) enterography/colonography. Contrast-enhanced ultrasound scanning (with Doppler) may also help to clarify the scenario but the quality of this test relies heavily on a high level of operator expertise [8]. Dynamic gadolinium-enhanced magnetic resonance imaging (MRI) and 18Ffluorodeoxyglucose positron emission tomography (FDG-PET) have also been shown to be excellent at highlighting active inflammation within a given stricture [10]. Diagnostic imaging also provides additional information on the length and complexity of any stricturing disease; characteristics that will also influence the management strategy in their own right. Direct endoscopic visualisation of a stricture and its surrounding mucosa is also a key part of the assessment process; endoscopic findings that strongly support active disease include the presence of marked mucosal ulceration and sloughing (Figure 2); endoscopic assessment also provides the opportunity to take biopsies for histopathological analysis. There is also an increased risk of malignancy in patients with stricturing or complex anorectal disease [11].

During the initial clinical work-up of patients who present with sub-acute symptoms associated with SB strictures, it is also important to consider the frequently overlooked co-existence of small intestinal bacterial overgrowth (SIBO) since treatment of this condition may have a significant impact on symptom alleviation [12].

Medical management

The acute or sub-acute symptomatic manifestation of a stricture is usually related to the plugging of the stenosis by indigestible dietary fibre or the presence of on-going mucosal oedema secondary to active inflammation. Unless the clinical scenario dictates otherwise, a conservative approach with medical and supportive therapy should be the first-line strategy. The response to medical therapy is, however, dependent on the inflammatory component within the stricture and strictures that are actively inflamed have a greater potential to respond to steroids and immunomodulatory agents than lesions that are already significantly fibrosed. Strictures that are likely to have a significant inflammatory component should therefore be managed with high-dose systemic steroids in the first instance; responders should then be maintained on long-term immunomodulators. Although the subject remains controversial, concerns regarding the potential for anti-tumour necrosis factor-α (anti-TNF-α) agents to worsen or induce fibrostenotic disease may be unfounded as the findings of several small series show [8, 13]. Adjusted multivariate analyses of patients included in the ACCENT I (A Crohn's Disease Clinical Trial Evaluating Infliximab in a New Long-Term Treatment Regimen) trial and the TREAT (the Crohn's Therapy, Resource, Evaluation, and Assessment Tool) registry showed that infliximab did not increase the likelihood of stenosis. On multivariate analysis, only disease duration, disease severity, terminal ileal disease and new corticosteroid use were associated with the development of strictures, stenosis and obstruction [4]. These data suggest that anti-TNF-α drugs may have a role to play in the management of active strictures that are refractory to initial treatment with steroids.

Endoscopic balloon dilatation

Since its introduction in the early 1980s, endoscopic balloon dilatation (EBD) has been shown to be a suitable alternative to surgery for selected patients with CD-related strictures. Most published series describing EBD relate to its use at colonoscopy for the management of ileocolic anastomotic, terminal ileal and colonic strictures. Long-term follow-up data from the largest such series published to date (138 patients, 237 dilatations) demonstrate that after a median follow-up of 5.8 years, 76% of patients avoided the need for surgery and only 46% required repeat EBD [14]. Since the recent advancement in deep enteroscopy techniques, EBD has become an option for SB strictures that were previously inaccessible to endoscopic therapy. Most data regarding EBD of strictures at deep enteroscopy come from work done with double-balloon enteroscopy (DBE) [15, 16] and outcomes for patients appear to be similar to EBD done at colonoscopy, leading to avoidance of surgery in a high proportion of appropriate patients [15, 16]. The outcomes of EBD are dependent on careful patient selection; short strictures (<5cm long) are more likely to have a favourable long-term response than longer ones [14-16]. EBD is associated with a 2-11% major complication rate, mainly in the form of bowel perforation. Factors such as endoscopic and EBD technique, quality of endoscopic views, which may be affected by bowel angulation at the site of stricture and the degree of active inflammation and ulceration affecting the targeted stricture, appear to play a significant role in the development of EBD-related complications [15]. The most frequently described EBD technique associated with successful outcomes involves the use of a through-the-scope (TTS) controlled radial expansion (CRE) balloon system (Boston Scientific Corp, Natick, MA, USA). Gradual inflation of the balloon with water under direct endoscopic vision to a maximum insufflation diameter of 18-20mm for 1-2 minutes is the generally recommended practice [14-16]. Careful radiological characterisation of the stricture before the EBD is contemplated, is often essential; this should also be combined with fluoroscopy for further evaluation of the stricture, at the time of EBD if possible. Maintenance of good long-term outcomes for EBD may require periodic re-dilatation as dictated by the symptom picture. Evidence to support the use of steroid injection into the stricture at the time of EBD is conflicting and this practice is not routinely recommended at present [14].

Surgical management

Although surgery is often unavoidable in the management of stricturing CD, it may be associated with significant morbidity and high postoperative recurrence rates. Up to 70% of patients develop endoscopic recurrence within 1 year of surgery and up to 40% of patients will be symptomatic again within 4 years [17]. Apart from the intrinsic risks associated with major surgery, patients undergoing repeated bowel resection for stricturing disease also face the hazard of short bowel syndrome. This has encouraged the development of surgical techniques such as strictureplasty in order to preserve SB length by minimising the need for bowel resection. The length of stenosis that can be repaired by strictureplasty is usually between 10 and 25cm [18]. The Heinecke-Mikulicz and Finney methods are the two most common techniques of strictureplasty performed in current practice. In the Heinecke-Mikulicz technique, a linear incision is made through the antimesenteric border of the stricture; this is extended by about 3cm on either side of the stricture and then sutured transversely with interrupted sutures in order to widen the SB lumen at the anastomosis. The Finney method is useful for longer strictures and involves the arrangement of the affected SB into a 'U'-shape, incising the stricture at the antimesenteric margin and closing this in a side-to-side fashion. A meta-analysis comparing these two methods, reported a lower re-operation rate in patients treated with the Finney method [19]. Traditionally, long strictures have been dealt with small bowel resection but in expert hands long strictureplasties (Michelassi) have been associated with good long-term success rates but can be associated with a higher rate of anastomotic leakage [20]. Strictureplasty is contraindicated in patients with on-going sepsis or in the presence of a fistula and is generally reserved for strictures involving the SB rather than the colon, since colonic strictures are deemed to be at higher risk of harbouring the potential for malignant transformation in longstanding CD of the colon [21].

Potential future management

Research into the use of candidate molecules that may arrest or reverse fibrogenesis hold promise to expand the future medical armamentarium available for this condition. Early work on removable self-expanding metal, plastic and biodegradable stent placement may also provide the foundations for additional alternative endoscopic options in the years to come.

Conclusions

Despite recent advances in the medical therapy of CD, the management of stricturing disease remains challenging. Although the immediate and long-term strategy will be dictated by the specific clinical scenario, as a general rule conservative measures should be explored first. The presence of on-going active inflammation within a strictured segment increases the likelihood of response to anti-inflammatory and immunomodulatory medication; however, fibrotic strictures will necessitate endoscopic or surgical intervention. Radiological and endoscopic evaluation should play a major role in the work-up of patients with stricturing CD; these investigations provide information about disease activity and anatomical characteristics that will decide the actual therapy. Short (<5cm) fibrotic strictures with favourable anatomic characteristics should be considered for EBD as an alternative to surgery. Patients who require surgical management for longer strictures that are not amenable to EBD should preferably be managed by bowel-conserving techniques such as strictureplasty in order to minimise the risk of inducing short bowel syndrome. A suggested management algorithm for stricturing CD is outlined in Figure 3.

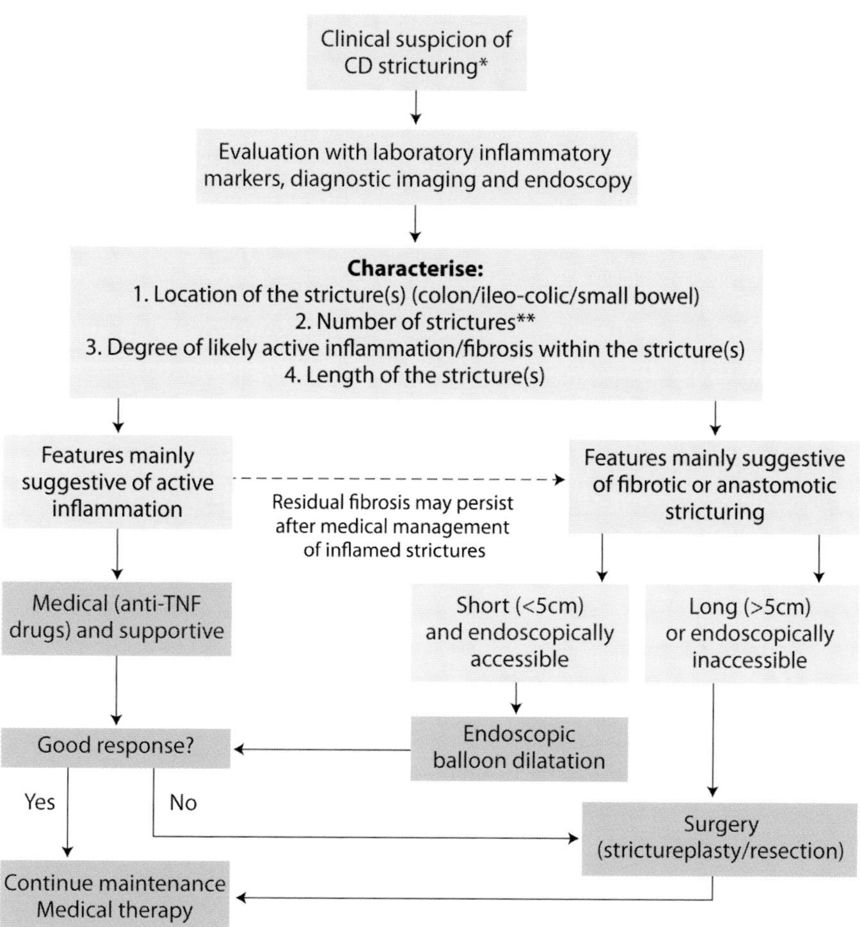

*consider ruling out superimposed small intestinal bacterial overgrowth (SIBO), as this may be contributing to symptoms
**may predispose to surgical management (strictureplasty/resection)

Figure 3. Suggested algorithm for the management of stricturing CD.

Key points

- **Crohn's disease (CD) is frequently complicated by the formation of strictures.**
- **Inflammatory strictures may respond to medical therapy but frequently strictures develop a significant fibrotic component that becomes refractory to medical therapy.**
- **Short (<5cm) fibrotic strictures respond well to endoscopic balloon dilatation (EBD) and in selected cases, this therapy may provide a lasting alternative to surgery.**
- **Strictures that are not amenable to EBD or have on-going active disease that is refractory to medical therapy frequently require surgical intervention.**
- **When surgery is required, bowel-conserving techniques such as strictureplasty should be employed if possible in order to minimise the risk of subsequent short bowel syndrome.**

References

1. Froehlich F, Juillerat P, Mottet C, *et al.* Obstructive fibrostenotic Crohn's disease. *Digestion* 2005; 71: 29-30.
2. Lahat A, Chowers Y. The patient with recurrent (sub) obstruction due to Crohn's disease. *Best Pract Res Clin Gastroenterol* 2007; 21: 427-44.
3. Alvarez-Lobos M, Arostegui JI, Sans M, *et al.* Crohn's disease patients carrying Nod2/CARD15 gene variants have an increased and early need for first surgery due to stricturing disease and higher rate of surgical recurrence. *Ann Surg* 2005; 242: 693-700.
4. Lichtenstein GR, Olson A, Travers S, *et al.* Factors associated with the development of intestinal strictures or obstructions in patients with Crohn's disease. *Am J Gastroenterol* 2006; 101: 1030-8.
5. Sands BE, Arsenault JE, Rosen MJ, *et al.* Risk of early surgery for Crohn's disease: implications for early treatment strategies. *Am J Gastroenterol* 2003; 98: 2712-8.
6. Louis E, Collard A, Oger AF, *et al.* Behaviour of Crohn's disease according to the Vienna classification: changing pattern over the course of the disease. *Gut* 2001; 49: 777-82.

7. Steson WF. Inflammatory bowel disease. In: *Yamada Textbook of Gastroenterology.* Yamada T, Alpers DH, Laine L, Owyang C, Powell DW, Eds. Philadelphia, USA: Lippincott Williams & Wilkins, 1999: 1775-839.
8. Sorrentino D. Role of biologics and other therapies in stricturing Crohn's disease: what have we learnt so far? *Digestion* 2008; 77: 38-47.
9. Florin TH, Paterson EW, Fowler EV, Radford-Smith GL. Clinically active Crohn's disease in the presence of a low C-reactive protein. *Scand J Gastroenterol* 2006; 41: 306-11.
10. Neurath MF, Vehling D, Schunk K, *et al.* Noninvasive assessment of Crohn's disease activity: a comparison of 18F-fluorodeoxyglucose positron emission tomography, hydromagnetic resonance imaging, and granulocyte scintigraphy with labeled antibodies. *Am J Gastroenterol* 2002; 97: 1978-85.
11. Connell WR, Sheffield JP, Kamm MA, *et al.* Lower gastrointestinal malignancy in Crohn's disease. *Gut* 1994; 35: 347-52.
12. Klaus J, Spaniol U, Adler G, *et al.* Small intestinal bacterial overgrowth mimicking acute flare as a pitfall in patients with Crohn's disease. *BMC Gastroenterol* 2009; 9: 61.
13. Pelletier AL, Kalisazan B, Wienckiewicz J, *et al.* Infliximab treatment for symptomatic Crohn's disease strictures. *Aliment Pharmacol Ther* 2009; 29: 279-85.
14. Thienpont C, D'Hoore A, Vermeire S, *et al.* Long-term outcome of endoscopic dilatation in patients with Crohn's disease is not affected by disease activity or medical therapy. *Gut* 2010; 59: 320-4.
15. Despott EJ, Gupta A, Burling D, *et al.* Effective dilation of small-bowel strictures by double-balloon enteroscopy in patients with symptomatic Crohn's disease (with video). *Gastrointest Endosc* 2009; 70: 1030-6.
16. Pohl J, May A, Nachbar L, Ell C. Diagnostic and therapeutic yield of push-and-pull enteroscopy for symptomatic small bowel Crohn's disease strictures. *Eur J Gastroenterol Hepatol* 2007; 19: 529-34.
17. Rutgeerts P, Geboes K, Vantrappen G, *et al.* Predictability of the postoperative course of Crohn's disease. *Gastroenterology* 1990; 99: 956-63.
18. Roy P, Kumar D. Strictureplasty. *Br J Surg* 2004; 91: 1428-37.
19. Tichansky D, Cagir B, Yoo E, *et al.* Strictureplasty for Crohn's disease: meta-analysis. *Dis Colon Rectum* 2000; 43: 911-9.
20. Michelassi F, Taschieri A, Tonelli F, *et al.* An international, multicenter, prospective, observational study of the side-to-side isoperistaltic strictureplasty in Crohn's disease. *Dis Colon Rectum* 2007; 50: 277-84.
21. Lukas M. Inflammatory bowel disease as a risk factor for colorectal cancer. *Dig Dis* 2010; 28: 619-24.

Chapter 12

Perianal fistula in Crohn's disease

Phil Tozer MBBS MRCS Eng MCEM Research Fellow, St Mark's Hospital, London, UK; Imperial College London, UK
Ailsa L. Hart BMBCh MRCP PhD Senior Clinical Lecturer, Imperial College and Consultant Gastroenterologist, St Mark's Hospital, London, UK
Siew Ng MBBS PhD MRCP Assistant Professor, Institute of Digestive Disease, Department of Medicine and Therapeutics, Chinese University of Hong Kong, Hong Kong; Senior Lecturer and Honorary Gastroenterologist, St Vincent's Hospital, University of Melbourne, Australia

Overview

Anal fistulae are common in Crohn's disease (CD), suggesting a severe disease course and are difficult to treat. Medical treatments such as antibiotics and immunosuppressants are the mainstay of treatment but suffer from slow onset, side effects and low remission and high recurrence rates. Recurrence and impairment of continence limit traditional surgical approaches. Combined medical and surgical treatment using anti-TNF agents in patients who undergo surgical drainage of sepsis with radiological monitoring of response provides rapid onset, robust healing in a third of patients and clinical benefit in the majority. An algorithm outlining this approach is shown below.

Introduction

Perianal fistulae are common in Crohn's disease (CD), occurring in around one in three patients over their lifetime [1]. They are unpleasant and difficult to treat, and are associated with a disabling disease course. Males, those with distal disease, a younger age of onset and non-Caucasian ethnicity are at a higher risk.

Historical series suggest the risk of proctectomy in patients with perianal fistulae in CD was as high as one in three [2] and that those complex fistulae which do heal take a median of 4 years and 6 interventions to do so [3].

Medical treatment has traditionally been with antibiotics, thiopurines and other immunomodulators, with surgery taking the form of faecal diversion or ablation (proctectomy). This approach is often largely palliative with little prospect of robust healing. Even proctectomy carries a one in three risk of delayed or failed perianal wound healing. Curative surgery on the fistula itself, for example, fistulotomy or advancement flap repair, has been less frequently undertaken and is less successful than in perianal fistulae of non-Crohn's origin.

The advent of anti-TNF agents has created the potential not only to improve quality of life but also to heal fistulae, and the time to clinical improvement has changed from the order of several months to a few weeks.

This improved treatment has prompted new questions: how to monitor patients, how long to treat them with anti-TNF agents and when, or perhaps if, to stop treatment. Serial imaging has emerged as a potential method for determining healing but further work is required to provide information on cessation of treatment as well as predictive factors which might limit exposure to anti-TNF agents in those patients who are unlikely to achieve remission.

The combination of biologic agents and surgery holds promise for the highest rates of anal fistula healing.

Assessment of perianal Crohn's disease

There are three ways to assess a patient with perianal CD besides history and physical examination:

- Endoscopy, for evaluating proximal luminal and, in particular, rectal disease.
- Local imaging with MRI or anal endosonography.
- Examination under anaesthesia with surgical drainage of any abscesses and seton placement as required.

These assessment methods are generally complementary and are often undertaken in combination. Endoscopy will assist in diagnosis and map the extent and severity of the known case. Additional small bowel imaging may be used to fully map the disease.

Pelvic MRI has been shown to be the most accurate method for classification of primary track and extensions [4], although anal ultrasound, particularly when enhanced by hydrogen peroxide, can occasionally be useful for detecting the internal opening where uncertainty exists. Anal ultrasound (in combination with anorectal physiology tests) can also assess sphincter integrity and function to inform an optimal surgical strategy. However, ultrasound will not reliably identify ischioanal fossa or supralevator sepsis due to rapidly declining resolution with distance from the probe. Furthermore, there is considerable variation in operator expertise and insertion of the ultrasound probe may be very uncomfortable in the setting of active sepsis, or impossible with stenosis.

On the other hand, MRI can be performed without a radiologist needing to be present at the time the test is done. Sequential images are easier to compare, particularly when monitoring treatment. Interpretation is more intuitive and the strategic view is better, which can be helpful intra-operatively. However, the test is expensive and the internal opening is less well seen (its position is usually inferred), and some patients feel claustrophobic in the confined space of the MRI scanner.

As well as being diagnostic, examination under anaesthetic (EUA) by an experienced surgeon allows infection to be drained and either definitive surgery (lay open or other curative procedures) or placement of a temporary loose seton for drainage while medical management is optimised. However, injudicious probing may cause iatrogenic tracks, increasing the complexity of the fistula and therefore the risk of recurrence or subsequent incontinence.

Treatment of perianal fistula in Crohn's disease (Table 1)

The established principles are to drain infection, use setons as required, aggressively manage active proctitis, give antibiotics, immunosuppressants, and employ anti-TNFα therapy, and they demand significant co-operation between gastroenterologists and surgeons.

Corticosteroids

Corticosteroids have no demonstrable role in perianal fistulae although they are sometimes used to treat concomitant luminal disease.

Metronidazole and ciprofloxacin

Both metronidazole and ciprofloxacin demonstrate a slow and incomplete response, early recurrence and unwanted side effects but often produce some symptomatic improvement.

Open-label studies with both drugs have shown improvement in most, if not all, patients, with remission in up to half, but relapse in three-quarters of these on cessation. A randomised trial found no benefit over placebo with either drug although numbers were small [5].

Overall, antibiotics remain a mainstay of treatment for perianal CD. If metronidazole is used, a dose of 750-1500mg/day is suggested. Adverse events include metallic taste, glossitis, nausea and neuropathy. It should be discontinued if any signs of neuropathy occur, but generally therapy is continued for 3-4 months. If ciprofloxacin is used, a dose of

Table 1. Medical treatment.

Drug	Study	Type of study	n	FU at endpoint	Fistula remission	
					Treatment	Placebo
Metronidazole	Thia 2009 [5]	RCT	7	10 weeks	0%	12.5%
Ciprofloxacin	Thia 2009 [5]	RCT	10	10 weeks	30%	12.5%
Aza/6-MP	Pearson 1995 [6]	Meta-analysis	41	-	*54%	*21%
Tacrolimus	Sandborn 2003 [18]	RCT	42	10 weeks	10%	8%
Infliximab	Present 1999 [7]	RCT induction	94	14 weeks	55%	13%
Infliximab	Accent II [8]	RCT maintenance	282	54 weeks	36%	19%
Adalimumab	CHARM # [13]	RCT maintenance	113	56 weeks	33%	13%

* = remission and response included together
\# = patients with luminal and perianal disease

500-1000mg/day is adequate and again is usually required for 3-4 months. Adverse events include headache, diarrhoea, nausea and rash.

Immunomodulators

There are no controlled trials which used a fistula as a primary outcome to support the use of azathioprine or 6-mercaptopurine (6-MP). Efficacy is suggested by a meta-analysis of trials which assessed fistulae as secondary endpoints and found a clinical fistula response of 54% (vs. 21% with placebo) [6]. A slow initial response, side effects and high recurrence rates mean durable fistula healing on thiopurines alone is unusual.

Inliximab

With the anti-TNF drugs comes a change in treatment options for perianal fistulating CD. The potential not only to improve quality of life but also to heal the fistula tracks has been realised and the time to clinical improvement has changed from the order of several months to a few weeks.

An early trial of 94 patients found a clinical response in 68% including remission in 50% with a response at a median of 2 weeks [7]. Maintenance therapy has been assessed in the ACCENT II trial (A Crohn's Disease Clinical Trial Evaluating Infliximab in a New Long-Term Treatment Regimen in Patients with Fistulizing Crohn's Disease) with 46% and 36% of responders in the treatment arm in response or remission, respectively, at 1 year (vs. 23% and 19% in the placebo group) [8]. Maintenance treatment reduced hospital admissions, length of stay and operations, and improved quality of life. On cessation, however, the risk of recurrence is higher than in luminal disease, with only 34% of patients free of relapse 1 year after cessation (vs. 83% in luminal disease) [9]. Concomitant thiopurines have not been shown to prevent relapse but may reduce perianal complications [10] and in luminal disease, steroid-free remission and mucosal healing are improved with dual therapy. The presence of proctitis predicts a poor response to infliximab and should be treated aggressively.

Infliximab and surgery

Examination under anaesthetic with drainage of trapped sepsis and insertion of setons where necessary, prior to commencement of infliximab therapy, improves the initial response to therapy and prevents or postpones recurrence [11]. There is also some evidence that pre-operative infliximab may improve outcome in surgery, although randomised trials are needed. A combined medical and surgical approach using anti-TNF agents in the surgically drained patient with radiological monitoring of response in a group of 41 patients has demonstrated rapid onset, robust healing in a third of patients and clinical benefit in the majority [12].

Adalimumab

Although no trials with adalimumab have evaluated fistula response or healing as a primary endpoint, in the CHARM (Crohn's trial of the fully Human Antibody Adalimumab for Remission Maintenance) study, 113 patients with Crohn's fistulae were given adalimumab at week 0 (80mg), week 2 (40mg) and then maintenance with either weekly or fortnightly adalimumab or placebo [13]. At 26 weeks, 30% of patients treated with adalimumab had complete closure and this rose to 33% at 56 weeks compared with 13% in the placebo arm. The CHARM study was extended for a further 2 years and a similar benefit was seen. Trials examining adalimumab efficacy after infliximab failure suggest a lower rate of remission but some patients do benefit from a second anti-TNF agent.

Monitoring response with MRI

After clinical healing (in the form of a closed external opening or cessation of drainage) on anti-TNF treatment has occurred, imaging modalities such as MRI indicate that the fistula track may remain for some time with deep and true healing of the fistula lagging behind clinical remission [14].

Early cessation of treatment prior to deep tissue healing may lead to early recurrence and radiological deterioration may indicate loss of response to the primary anti-TNF agent used. The use of serial imaging has been suggested to help delineate the appropriate time to alter treatment either because healing has occurred or because a change in dose or drug is required to recapture response. Imaging may also indicate the need for further surgical intervention during maintenance treatment to drain abscesses or place setons. Studies utilising MRI to monitor response to anti-TNF treatment have indicated that radiological healing lags behind clinical remission by a median of 12 months and that long-term maintenance treatment may be required to prevent recurrence in spite of a clinically healed external opening [12]. The search for clinical and radiological factors which predict ultimate failure and success of anti-TNF treatment is underway.

Surgery (Tables 2 and 3)

The surgeon's role in Crohn's perianal fistulae has changed and management is now performed in combination with the physician. Some fistulae can be definitively cured surgically, usually by a lay open or advancement flap technique (Table 2), whilst other patients need palliation

Table 2. Curative surgery.

A few patients with moderate Crohn's disease may be candidates for curative surgery:

- Advancement flap (good rectum, perineal descent/internal intussusception helpful, consider temporary stoma)
- Coloanal pull through (rectal internal opening, good anus, good colon, loop ileostomy)
- Turnbull-Cutait (internal opening at dentate line, good anus, good colon, loop ileostomy)
- Fistulotomy +/- delayed sphincter repair (consider temporary stoma)

Some patients with severe and debilitating disease may benefit from ablative surgery.

of their symptoms or even a proctectomy (Table 3). Palliation usually comes in the form of drainage of any trapped infection and thereafter a long-term, comfortable loose seton.

Examination under anaesthetic, drainage of sepsis and insertion of comfortable setons now forms the first stage in the truly combined surgical-medical treatment of anal fistulae using infliximab as described above. If pre-treatment surgical drainage is inadequate, abscess formation during the infliximab course may be more likely and can cause the treatment to fail.

Fistulotomy is used sparingly in Crohn's anal fistulae because of concerns regarding future fistula formation and problems with healing, and also because increased bowel frequency and the tendency for this to worsen with disease activity or future resection makes incontinence a greater threat.

Advancement flaps can be used as a sphincter-preserving technique for some higher fistulae in CD with a success rate of around 50% and are appropriate in those who do not have active proctitis or extensive cavitating ulceration in the anal canal. A defunctioning stoma is sometimes

Table 3. Ablative surgery.

Perianal fistulae alone are unlikely to lead to very poor general health with restriction of work or social activities; colorectal disease is likely to be to blame. In this case:

- Medical management should be optimised
- If this fails, proctectomy or proctocolectomy (dependent on the extent of disease) should be considered
- Advice regarding the risk of delayed or poor perineal wound healing should be given

used in an attempt to improve the chance of success, although there is little evidence to support this. Fistula glues and plugs have been examined in small trials of Crohn's patients and although randomised data are needed to demonstrate their efficacy they present little risk to the sphincter complex or future success with alternative treatment. Palliation through permanent seton insertion or ablation with proctectomy (+/- colectomy) may be necessary and lead to an improved quality of life. Proctectomy carries risks of luminal recurrence, reoperation, damage to pelvic nerves and a delayed or unhealed perineal wound, but may provide significant relief where severe proctitis and perianal disease have affected the patient's life. It may still be needed in around 10% of patients [15]. Defunctioning alone has little long-term benefit and often leads to permanent diversion [16].

Algorithm

An algorithm for the approach and management of perianal Crohn's fistula is outlined in Figure 1, in which aggressive management of both luminal and perianal disease is recommended with close co-operation between surgeons, radiologists and gastroenterologists [17].

Conclusions

Crohn's anal fistulae are unpleasant, difficult to treat and common. The associated disease course is often severe and disabling, and multiple medical and surgical interventions are often required. Combined surgical and medical treatment using combination therapy with antibiotics, thiopurines and anti-TNF agents, adequate initial and, where necessary, repeated surgical drainage and radiological monitoring of response is emerging as the most effective mode of treatment.

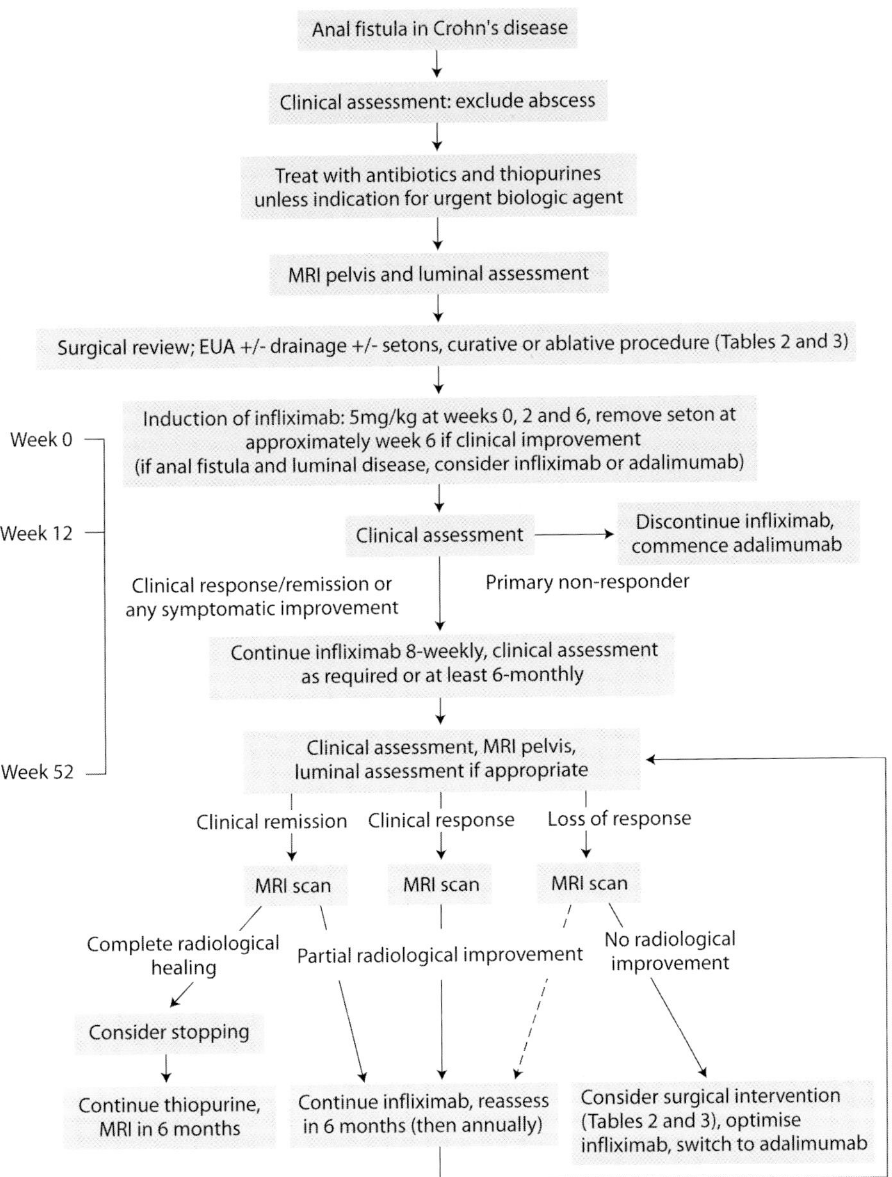

Figure 1. Algorithm for the management of anal fistulae in Crohn's disease.

Key points

- **Perianal fistulae are common in Crohn's disease and suggest a severe disease course.**
- **Careful assessment of perianal Crohn's disease is needed with radiological techniques such as MRI or endoanal ultrasound and examination under anaesthesia.**
- **Perianal disease needs to be considered in the context of disease elsewhere in the gastrointestinal tract.**
- **Antibiotics (metronidazole and ciprofloxacin), thiopurines and anti-TNF drugs form the mainstay of medical treatment.**
- **Adequate surgical drainage of trapped sepsis +/- seton insertion is needed before commencement of anti-TNF therapy.**
- **Combined medical and surgical treatment with radiological monitoring of response provides optimal outcomes.**

References

1. Ardizzone S, Porro GB. Perianal Crohn's disease: overview. *Dig Liver Dis* 2007; 39: 957-8.
2. Hellers G, Bergstrand O, Ewerth S, Holmstrom B. Occurrence and outcome after primary treatment of anal fistulae in Crohn's disease. *Gut* 1980; 21: 525-7.
3. Bell SJ, Williams AB, Wiesel P *et al.* The clinical course of fistulating Crohn's disease. *Aliment Pharmacol Ther* 2003; 17: 1145-51.
4. Sahni VA, Ahmad R, Burling D. Which method is best for imaging of perianal fistula? *Abdom Imaging* 2008; 33: 26-30.
5. Thia KT, Mahadevan U, Feagan BG, *et al.* Ciprofloxacin or metronidazole for the treatment of perianal fistulae in patients with Crohn's disease: a randomized, double-blind, placebo-controlled pilot study. *Inflamm Bowel Dis* 2009; 15: 17-24.
6. Pearson DC, May GR, Fick GH, Sutherland LR. Azathioprine and 6-mercaptopurine in Crohn disease. A meta-analysis. *Ann Intern Med* 1995; 123: 132-42.
7. Present DH, Rutgeerts P, Targan S, *et al.* Infliximab for the treatment of fistulae in patients with Crohn's disease. *N Engl J Med* 1999; 340(18): 1398-405.
8. Sands BE, Anderson FH, Bernstein CN, *et al.* Infliximab maintenance therapy for fistulizing Crohn's disease. *N Engl J Med* 2004; 350: 876-85.

9. Domenech E, Hinojosa J, Nos P, *et al.* Clinical evolution of luminal and perianal Crohn's disease after inducing remission with infliximab: how long should patients be treated? *Aliment Pharmacol Ther* 2005; 22: 1107-13.
10. Sokol H, Seksik P, Carrat F, *et al.* Usefulness of co-treatment with immunomodulators in patients with inflammatory bowel disease treated with scheduled infliximab maintenance therapy. *Gut* 2010; 59: 1363-8.
11. Regueiro M, Mardini H. Treatment of perianal fistulizing Crohn's disease with infliximab alone or as an adjunct to exam under anesthesia with seton placement. *Inflamm Bowel Dis* 2003; 9: 98-103.
12. Tozer PJ, Ng SC, Siddiqui MR, *et al.* Long-term MRI-guided combined anti-TNFα and thiopurine therapy for Crohn's perianal fistulas. *Inflamm Bowel Dis* 2011: in press.
13. Colombel JF, Sandborn WJ, Rutgeerts P, *et al.* Adalimumab for maintenance of clinical response and remission in patients with Crohn's disease: the CHARM trial. *Gastroenterology* 2007; 132: 52-65.
14. Ng SC, Plamondon S, Gupta A, *et al.* Prospective evaluation of anti-tumor necrosis factor therapy guided by magnetic resonance imaging for Crohn's perineal fistulae. *Am J Gastroenterol* 2009; 104(12): 2973-86.
15. Gaertner WB, Decanini A, Mellgren A, *et al.* Does infliximab infusion impact results of operative treatment for Crohn's perianal fistulae? *Dis Colon Rectum* 2007; 50(11): 1754-60.
16. Yamamoto T, Allan RN, Keighley MR. Effect of fecal diversion alone on perianal Crohn's disease. *World J Surg* 2000; 24: 1258-62.
17. Tozer PJ, Burling D, Gupta A, *et al.* Review article: medical, surgical and radiological management of perianal Crohn's fistulae. *Aliment Pharmacol Ther* 2011; 33: 5-22.
18. Sandborn WJ, Present DH, Isaacs KL, *et al.* Tacrolimus for the treatment of fistulae in patients with Crohn's disease: a randomized, placebo-controlled trial. *Gastroenterology* 2003; 125: 380-8.

Chapter 13

Fistulating non-perianal Crohn's disease

Cheng T. Tee MB BCh BAO MRCP(UK)(Gastroenterology) Research Fellow, St Mark's Hospital, London, UK

Carolynne Vaizey MBChB MD FRCS(Gen) FCS(SA) Consultant Colorectal Surgeon, St Mark's Hospital, London, UK

Jeremy Nightingale MB BS FRCP MD Cert MHS Consultant in Gastroenterology and Nutritional Support, St Mark's Hospital, London, UK

Simon M. Gabe MD MSc BSc MBBS FRCP Consultant Gastroenterologist, St Mark's Hospital, London, UK

Overview

Fistulating non-perianal Crohn's disease (CD) is a complex and difficult to treat complication of CD that can lead to significant physical and psychosocial distress for patients. General principles of fistulae management include the immediate treatment and control of sepsis (identifying and draining intra-abdominal collections), correction of fluid and electrolyte disturbances, pain management and early wound management. Once these factors have been addressed, nutritional support may be given (via enteral or parenteral route) and tighter control of the fistula output may help towards early spontaneous closure of fistulae. Defining the anatomy is helpful in establishing the likelihood of spontaneous closure and in planning surgical procedures. Surgical removal of a fistula and re-establishment of bowel continuity is delayed till at least 4 months after the fistula first appeared. Treatment with antibiotics, thiopurines and anti-TNF agents may improve spontaneous closure rates of fistulae in CD. Cyclosporine and tacrolimus should be used only when other drugs are unsuccessful. A multidisciplinary approach contributes to optimal treatment and improved patient quality of life.

Introduction

Crohn's disease (CD) is a chronic inflammatory bowel disease (IBD) typified by transmural inflammation, anywhere from the mouth to the anus, which can lead to the development of fistulae during the course of the disease. Population-based studies have estimated that the cumulative incidence of fistulae in CD is 33% after 10 years from diagnosis and 50% after 20 years. Of these, 54% were perianal, 24% were enteroenteric, 9% were rectovaginal and 13% were classified as 'other' type [1]. One third of these patients had recurrent fistulae.

The natural history is one of exacerbations, lengthy healing and protracted episodes of actively draining fistulae. The classification of fistulae is based on their location and connection with contiguous organs (Figure 1).

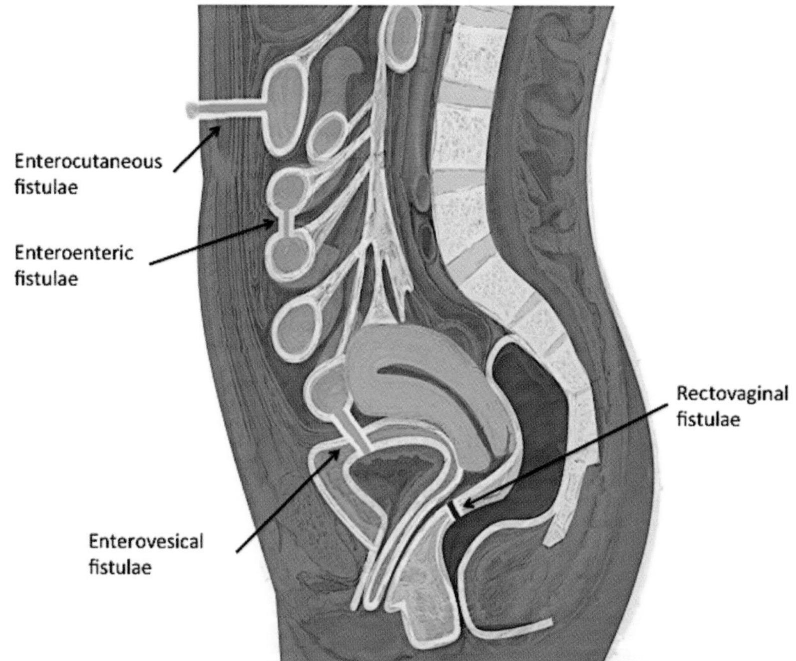

Figure 1. Classification of fistulae based on location and connection with contiguous organs.

Traditionally, fistulae have been associated with a high risk of morbidity and death related to sepsis, malnutrition and fluid, electrolyte or metabolic disturbances. Mortality rates for non-CD enterocutaneous fistulae (ECF) have, however, improved from 44% to approximately 15% between the 1940s and 1970s [2], with a further decrease to 5% in 2010 [3]. Whether this is similar in the subgroup of CD patients is unknown. However, more favourable outcomes are associated with a multidisciplinary approach to control sepsis early, address nutritional support, define the intestinal anatomy and time appropriate surgery, if required. Members of the multidisciplinary team are listed in Table 1.

Table 1. Multidisciplinary team involved in the care of patients with Crohn's disease fistula.

- Nutrition support team (NST):

  - gastroenterologist (usually heads the team)
  - specialist nutrition nurse
  - dietition
  - pharmacist

- Radiologist
- Gastrointestinal surgeon (gynaecologist, urologist, plastic surgeon)
- Chemical pathologist
- Microbiologist
- Stoma care nurse/tissue viability nurse
- Pain management team
- Psychiatrist
- Physiotherapist
- Occupational therapist
- Social worker

In this chapter we discuss the general management options available to treat CD fistulae based on current experience and evidence. Some of the basic principles are shared with non-CD fistulae management. Much of the published evidence on fistulising CD deals with the management of perianal fistula whereas data on the management of internal fistulae are scarce. The available literature has been largely derived from retrospective series, mostly from large specialist centres with expertise in the management of this condition. However, the general principles of management can be applied to all fistulae. The specific management of perianal Crohn's fistulae has been covered in Chapter 12.

The medical and surgical approach to managing fistulising Crohn's disease (Figure 2)

The traditional approach of a patient who has developed an intestinal fistula was to place the patient on total parenteral nutrition (TPN) (nil by mouth [NBM] and parenteral nutrition [PN]) and a somatostatin or somatostatin analogue. There is, however, increasing evidence to suggest that oral and/or enteral nutrition together with appropriate management of sepsis is as effective as the traditional approach. Traditional teaching of the SNAP approach (Sepsis, Nutrition, define Anatomy and Plan surgery) has previously helped physicians in focusing on the important issues during fistulae management, but there is much more to consider than just those four principles. Current principles of managing an intestinal fistula should be divided into immediate, early and late management, as outlined below.

Immediate – sepsis

Sepsis is common in patients with fistulae and rapid aggressive treatment with broad-spectrum intravenous antibiotics (guided by culture sensitivity) and appropriate fluid resuscitation is required [4, 5]. In the first hours of presentation particular attention should be given to volume restoration and correction of electrolyte imbalance. Losses from high-output fistulae should be assessed and replaced every 4 hours.

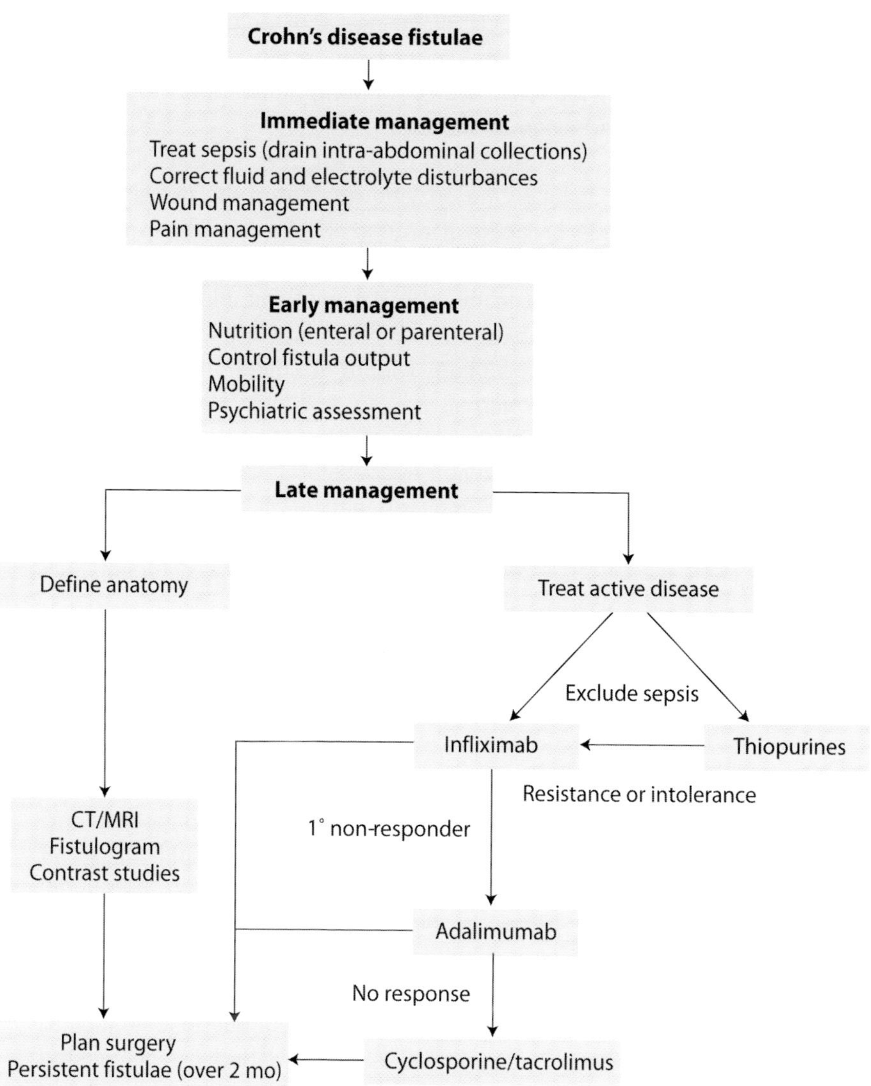

Figure 2. Algorithm for internal and EC fistula.

In addition, it is important to ascertain if the patient has any intra-abdominal sepsis with discrete collections. This will require appropriate imaging (usually ultrasound or CT scanning) and radiological drainage. Surgical drainage is usually not necessary apart from exceptional circumstances as collections are commonly amenable to CT or ultrasonographic-guided external drainage.

In terms of external fistulae, the enzyme content of the fistula effluent can lead to rapid tissue breakdown around the fistula, which prevents spontaneous closure and predisposes to infection. Therefore, skin protection should be tailored to the specific anatomic circumstances of each fistula. A skilled dedicated nurse or enterostomal therapist capable of fashioning the effluent collection system to meet the unique and changing needs of each wound is key to success. Vacuum-assisted wound management can be helpful but must be kept away from the bowel as it can itself induce a fistula. When successful, these systems reduce the need for dressing changes and can accelerate fistula closure by promoting wound healing [6]. From a medical perspective, these issues can be easily overlooked but from the patient's viewpoint they may be the most important.

Early – nutrition

Effective nutrition can be only delivered when a patient is not septic and fluid balance has been achieved; therefore, in the immediate situation it is reasonable to withhold all nutrition (including parenteral nutrition). Once the sepsis and fluid imbalance is controlled, early nutritional supplementation should be addressed to avoid a patient becoming malnourished. Multiple factors contribute to this and include a limited supply of nutrients (due to anorexia or restriction of oral intake), loss of protein, electrolytes and fluids from the fistula effluent due to loss of small bowel secretions that would ordinarily be reabsorbed, and loss of ingested nutrients due to high output fistulae. Also, there is an increased demand for energy as a result of sepsis and inflammation. There is a significantly higher incidence of complications and higher mortality rates in malnourished patients undergoing abdominal surgery for both benign and malignant gastrointestinal disease [7, 8].

Opinions differ in terms of the best route of administration. The concept of 'bowel rest' with the use of TPN is based on two beliefs: firstly, that food is a culture medium and if leaking into the peritoneal cavity it is likely to promote sepsis and, secondly, the observation that gastrointestinal secretions fall by 30-50% in patients receiving TPN [9], which may aid fistula closure. However, despite a decrease in fistula output there may not be a significant effect on fistula closure [3]. There are currently no randomised trials investigating outcomes of patients kept NBM [10] and in a series of 1168 ECF patients reported by Li *et al* [11], only 13.6% of the patients received PN exclusively, yet mortality was very low and overall closure rates were high. This suggests that oral/enteral feeding may reduce fistula output and promote closure as effectively as TPN [12]. In support for enteral feeding, critical care literature suggests that enteral nutrition is superior to PN in intensive care and postoperative settings. A recent meta-analysis demonstrated a reduced incidence of infection in patients requiring intensive care who received enteral rather than PN, although overall mortality was not different [13]. Considering that extended periods of NBM is very difficult for a patient psychologically, many centres are now allowing patients to have oral/enteral nutrition early.

Oral/enteral feeding should be appropriate if a fistula is draining directly from the bowel to the skin or into a shallow wound (as occurs in the most common midline postoperative enterocutaneous fistulae) and if there is sufficient bowel proximal to the fistula for absorption (more than 100cm). If the bowel contents leak into the peritoneal cavity and are associated with an abscess cavity and a long fistula tract, it may be wise to rest the gut until the situation stabilises. In time the fistula tract will become shorter and the associated intra-abdominal sepsis will resolve making oral/enteral feeding possible.

Manipulation of fistula output is important at this stage. It reduces the volume of irritant effluent in external fistulae, which facilitates improved skin care. Patients with high fistula output (>2L/day) will have significant fluid and electrolyte losses (in general 100mmol sodium in a litre of small bowel fistula output) that need to be replaced parenterally. Reduction of fistula output can be achieved by adopting a high-output ileostomy/jejunostomy regimen. This involves fluid restriction, using an electrolyte mix orally, antimotility agents (loperamide and codeine phosphate) and in most, antisecretory drugs (proton pump inhibitors and occasionally octreotide) [14, 15]. Somatostatin has a dramatic effect on reducing fistula output, but its clinical use is limited by the short half-life of 1-3 minutes. The synthetic analogue octreotide has a half-life of 90 minutes and reduces all GI secretions, prolongs gastric and small bowel transit times and facilitates absorption of water and electrolytes [16]. Comparisons between somatostatin and octreotide have shown somatostatin to be more effective in reducing fistula output than octreotide [10]. There is very little evidence to suggest that either agent increases the overall likelihood of spontaneous fistula closure and there are no data on the CD subset of patients.

Early mobility with physiotherapy is important to prevent contractures and muscle wasting which will aid in early discharge. Patients often find themselves isolated dealing with the complexities of Crohn's disease and fistulae complications that may lead to a range of overt and covert manifestations of emotional distress. An early supportive framework in the form of counselling and psychotherapy will help patients cope with their illness and contribute to a better quality of life.

Late – define anatomy

The correct anatomical identification of a fistula is essential to enable the clinician to select the most appropriate therapy. This information is used to assess the likelihood of spontaneous closure and inadequate delineation can lead to potential poor clinical outcomes and misclassification of simple fistulae may result in progression to complex forms. Physicians should suspect ongoing sepsis from an abscess when a patient is not putting on weight despite nutritional support, has evidence of active inflammation (a high white cell and platelet count, a high C-reactive protein level and a low albumin level) and spiking temperatures.

The available diagnostic modalities include computed tomography (CT), pelvic magnetic resonance imaging (MRI) or MR enterography, contrast follow-through studies and anorectal ultrasound. When any of the two diagnostic modalities are used in combination, an accuracy of 100% can be achieved in defining the exact anatomy [17].

Late – plan surgery

The goal in fistula management is fistula closure with minimal morbidity and mortality. Rates of spontaneous fistula closure in non-CD patients range from 19% [18] to 92% [19], although the upper extremes reflect small studies with selected subgroups of patients. Spontaneous closure rates of non-CD ECF have been reported to be as low as 20% in 277 patients treated between 1992 and 2002 at St Mark's Hospital [20] in contrast to higher spontaneous closure rates of 75% in 147 treated in Durban between 1990 and 1999 [21]. Therefore, the range in spontaneous closure rates suggests a difference in patient population and ECF characteristics. Factors that favour spontaneous fistula closure are shown in Table 2.

Table 2. Factors that favour spontaneous fistula closure [9, 22].

- Surgical aetiology
- Free distal flow (no distal obstruction)
- Healthy surrounding bowel
- Simple fistula with no associated abscess cavity
- Fistula tract >2cm
- Fistula tract not epithelialised
- Enteral defect <1cm (with no discontinuity)
- Low fistula output
- No external visible bowel mucosa
- No comorbidity

If the fistula remains open after 2 months, surgical intervention is likely to be needed as spontaneous closure is unlikely after this interval [23]. ECF are unlikely to heal without surgery if there is mucocutaneous discontinuity, ongoing disease or sepsis of the fistula site, visible gut mucosa, distal obstruction and multiple fistulae. Timing of corrective surgery is important and should be planned early. However, delayed surgery is recommended. This is because early major abdominal surgery, between 10-100 days will be difficult as the bowel is friable and will easily tear, therefore increasing the risk of fistula formation; it will also stimulate dense adhesions especially when complicated by intra-abdominal sepsis [24, 25]. Delayed surgery will also allow metabolic and nutritional deficiencies to be corrected.

Drug treatment for fistulising Crohn's disease (Table 3)

Data from placebo-controlled clinical trials investigating the use of 6-mercaptopurine, tacrolimus and infliximab have shown that approximately 10% of patients with fistulising CD achieved spontaneous fistula healing on placebo treatment. This low spontaneous healing rate suggests that combined approaches with medical and possible surgical interventions are often required.

Corticosteroids and 5-aminosalicylate acid

Corticosteroids are effective for the treatment of active luminal CD, but in patients with Crohn's fistulae, prednisolone has been shown in three studies (two large uncontrolled, one case-controlled) to have more detrimental outcomes in the form of increased surgical intervention and abscesses compared with patients not on steroids [26]. Corticosteroids should therefore be used sparingly when there are no signs of active luminal inflammation and when one is dealing solely with fistulae.

There are no clinical data to date that show a beneficial effect of mesalazine on fistula healing.

Antibiotics

Although not proven, it has been suggested that bacteria play a role in the pathogenesis of fistula formation. Antibiotics in the form of metronidazole and ciprofloxacin have been traditionally used as first-line medical therapy for perianal Crohn's fistulae with some studies reporting a closure rate of up to 50% in perianal fistulae. However, they only provide short-term benefits as up to 78% of patients had symptomatic recurrence within 4 months of stopping. Also, side effects associated with both antibiotics in the form of dyspepsia, disulfiram-like response to alcohol, peripheral neuropathy and paraesthesia, headaches, diarrhoea and rash limits their use [27]. There are no controlled data using antibiotics for treatment of internal fistulae.

Apart from antibiotics being used as primary therapy in fistulae, they are also commonly used as an adjuvant therapy for abscesses and infections caused by fistulae. More often of late, antibiotics are used as a bridge before azathioprine takes effect. However, when used in combination with infliximab, it has been shown that the primary outcomes of perianal fistula healing was not improved by the addition of ciprofloxacin to infliximab compared to infliximab alone [28].

Thiopurines

Azathioprine and 6-mercaptopurine (MP) are immunosuppressive agents shown to be effective in treating luminal inflammation in CD. There are no controlled trials using these two agents with fistula healing as primary endpoints. A meta-analysis of five randomised controlled trials with closure of various fistulae (including perianal, enterocutaneous, enteroenteric, rectovaginal and vulva types) as a secondary endpoint showed a beneficial effect of azathioprine and MP in 54% of patients compared to 21% in those receiving placebo [29]. Thiopurines can therefore be used as a second-line treatment of fistulae that are not in need of immediate surgery in conjunction with antibiotics.

Calcineurin inhibitors

There are no controlled data supporting the use of calcineurin inhibitors in fistulising CD. Case series have, however, shown that cyclosporine administered intravenously may have a role in the treatment of fistulae especially in the acute setting. In one study, nine out of the ten patients with fistulising CD that did not respond to azathioprine or MP responded well to cyclosporine [30]. In the largest case series to date, 88% of patients with fistulising disease had an initial response to intravenous cyclosporine; seven out of ten patients achieved complete closure of their fistulae [31].

In a randomised, double-blinded, placebo-controlled, multicenter study involving 48 patients with fistulising CD, 43% of the tacrolimus-treated patients had fistula improvement compared with 8% in the placebo group; the remission rate was comparable between both groups (10% vs. 8%, respectively) [32]. More patients who had tacrolimus had serious adverse events.

Both cyclosporine and tacrolimus are reserved for when other treatments have been unsuccessful.

Anti-tumour necrosis factor agents

The efficacy of infliximab in the treatment of patients with fistulising CD was demonstrated in a randomised, multicentre, double-blind, placebo-controlled trial. There were a total of nine enterocutaneous and 85 perianal fistula patients. Patients were randomly assigned to infliximab (5mg/kg or 10mg/kg) or placebo at 0, 2 and 6 weeks. The primary endpoint was at least 50% reduction from baseline in the number of draining fistulae on at least two consecutive assessments. Approximately 62% of the patients in either infliximab group (5mg/kg and 10mg/kg) achieved the primary endpoint of the study compared with 26% of those in the placebo group (p=0.002). There was no difference in response rates between both infliximab groups. Complete fistulae closure occurred in 46% of those receiving infliximab compared to 13% of those on placebo (p=0.001). The median time to response was 2 weeks and the median length of time during which the fistulae remained closed was 3 months [33].

Table 3. Summary of evidence for pharmacological treatment options in fistulising Crohn's disease. *Adapted from Vavricka SR, et al* [39].

Author	Drug	Study period	Study type	Outcome
Antibiotics				
Bernstein 1980 [27]	Metro	10 weeks	Open label	Clinical response (21/21) within 8 weeks; 56% (10/18) complete healing
West 2004 [28]	Cipro +IFX	18 weeks	RCT	>50% reduction in draining fistula: 73% (8/11) cipro + IFX vs. 39% (5/13) IFX alone
Immuno-suppressive agents				
Pearson 1995 [29]	6-MP, AZA	N/A	Meta-analysis 5 trials	Response rate (a decrease in discharge): 54% (22/41) AZA/6-MP vs. 21% (6/29) placebo
Egan 1998 [30]	Cyclo	Up to 22 weeks	Retrospective	77% (7/9) partial response
Present 1994 [31]	Cyclo	Up to 37 months	Open label	88% (14/16) initial response; 44% (7/16) complete healing
Sandborn 2003 [32]	Tacro	10 weeks	RCT	>50% reduction in draining fistula Improvement: 43% (9/21) tacro vs. 8% (2/25) placebo; complete healing: 10% (2/21) tacro vs. 8% (2/25) placebo
Anti-TNF agents				
Present 1999 [33]	IFX	18 weeks	RCT	>50% reduction in draining fistula: 62% (39/62) IFX vs. 26% (8/31) placebo Complete healing: 46% (29/63) IFX vs. 13% (4/31) placebo
Sands 2004 [34]	IFX	54 weeks	RCT	50% reduction in draining fistula: 46% (42/91) IFX vs. 23% (23/98) placebo Complete healing: 36% (33/91) IFX vs. 19% (19/98) placebo
Colombel 2007 [35]	Ada	56 weeks	RCT	Complete healing: 33% (23/70) ada vs. 13% (6/47) placebo

All randomised controlled trials (RCT) were double-blind and placebo-controlled. Metro = metronidazole; Cipro = ciprofloxacin; Aza = azathioprine; 6-MP = 6-mercaptopurine; Cyclo = cyclosporine A; Tacro = Tacrolimus; IFX = infliximab; Ada = adalimumab.

The ACCENT II trial evaluated the efficacy of repeated infusions of infliximab in maintaining closure of draining fistulae among those who had previously responded to infliximab. Of 282 patients who had a minimum of a 3-month duration of perianal or enterocutaneous fistula (10% of patients) treated with 5mg/kg infliximab at 0, 2 and 6 weeks, 69% responded. The responders were then randomised to receive infliximab or placebo at 8-week intervals until week 54. The median time to loss of response to treatment was significantly longer in the infliximab group (40 weeks versus 14 weeks). After the 54 weeks, 46% of the infliximab group had a sustained response compared to 23% in the placebo group. A post hoc analysis of the results in 27 women with rectovaginal fistulae showed that approximately 64% of patients achieved fistula closure when treated with infliximab; those who received maintenance therapy had a more durable response compared to those on placebo. Secondary analysis showed that maintenance therapy with infliximab resulted in significantly lower rates of hospitalisation and a reduced need for surgeries and procedures including total parenteral nutrition [34].

Patients intolerant to infliximab or who experienced loss of response to infliximab should be offered adalimumab induction and maintenance. The CHARM study assessed fistula closure as a secondary endpoint. In the subgroup of 117 infliximab-naïve and infliximab-exposed patients with fistulising CD, adalimumab was associated with improved fistula closure at week 26 (30% vs. 13%; p=0.043) and week 56 (33% vs. 13%; p=0.016) when compared with placebo. The recommended induction subcutaneous dose of adalimumab is 160mg with a second dose of 80mg during week 2 and the maintenance dose is 40mg every other week after week 4. If there is loss of response, a weekly dose is recommended [35].

Continuous certolizumab treatment can also increase the likelihood of sustained fistulae closure. In patients who responded to 6 weeks of certolizumab, 36% of patients in the certolizumab pegol group had 100% fistula closure compared with 17% of patients receiving placebo at week 26. The majority of patients in this study had perianal fistula (55 of 58) [36].

Three doses of infliximab therapy followed by continued use of azathioprine or MP may achieve persistent fistula closure. In an open-label study, 16 patients with fistulising CD were treated with three or four infliximab infusions and long-term azathioprine or MP; 75% of patients had complete fistula closure persisting for at least 6 months [37]. These patients were thiopurine-naïve.

Whilst anti-TNF agents may be an appropriate therapy for fistulising disease, they can be associated with an increased risk of malignancies, immunological reactions and infections. In two clinical trials, 11% and 15% patients developed abscesses related to their fistulae whilst on infliximab; however, it is unclear whether this rate is higher than the spontaneous rate of abscess formation in patients with fistulae [33, 38]. Therefore, clearance of sepsis via drainage before initiating anti-TNF agents would be best practice.

Other treatments

Case studies and retrospective reviews have shown some modest efficacy of methotrexate, mycophenolate mofetil, thalidomide or octreotide in the management of fistulising CD. Other experimental methods include the use of granulocyte macrophage colony-stimulating factor (GM-CSF) and hyperbaric oxygen.

Conclusions

Fistulising Crohn's disease can lead to significant physical and psychosocial distress for patients, and despite available medical, surgical and pharmacological treatment, the chance of complete healing is less than 50%. The control of sepsis, wound management and nutritional support alongside a multidisciplinary team may lead to better outcomes. Antibiotics, azathioprine/6-mercaptopurine may heal fistulae in up to 50% of cases. Once sepsis has been excluded with imaging and clinical assessment, anti-TNF agents can be considered although there are limited data on long-term outcome of their efficacy in non-perianal fistulae. Cyclosporine and tacrolimus may be considered. Planned surgical intervention is likely if spontaneous closure of the fistulae has not occurred after 2 months.

Key points

- Fistulising Crohn's disease is associated with a high risk of morbidity and death related to sepsis, malnutrition and fluid and electrolyte disturbances.
- The general principles of management are divided into immediate, early and late management:
  - o Immediate:
    - intra-abdominal sepsis identified and drained (+/- antibiotics);
    - water and electrolyte disturbances corrected;
    - good wound management;
    - pain control.
  - o Early:
    - initiate nutritional support (enteral or parenteral route);
    - control fistula output;
    - psychosocial assessment;
    - mobility.
  - o Late:
    - anatomy defined to establish chance of spontaneous closure of fistula, assess gut length and quality;
    - planned surgery but avoid day 10-100, giving the fistula time to close spontaneously (at least 2 months).
- Drug treatment includes using antibiotics, thiopurines and anti-TNF agents. Cyclosporine and tacrolimus are reserved for when other drugs fail.
- A multidisciplinary team is essential in providing co-ordinated care with low mortality and morbidity rates.

References

1. Schwartz DA, Loftus EV, Tremaine WJ, *et al.* The natural history of fistulizing Crohn's disease in Olmsted County, Minnesota. *Gastroenterology* 2002; 122: 875-80.

2. Soeters PB, Ebeid AM, Fischer JE. Review of 404 patients with gastrointestinal fistulas. Impact of parenteral nutrition. *Ann Surg* 1979; 190: 189-202.
3. Mawdsley JE, Hollington, Bassett PP, *et al.* An analysis of predictive factors for healing and mortality in patients with enterocutaneous fistulas. *Aliment Pharmacol Ther* 2008; 28: 1111-21.
4. Allardyce DB. Management of small bowel fistulas. *Am J Surg* 1983; 145: 593-5.
5. Rolandelli R, Roslyn JJ. Surgical management and treatment of sepsis associated with gastrointestinal fistulas. *Surg Clin North Am* 1996; 76: 1111-22.
6. Banwell P, Withey S, Holten I. The use of negative pressure to promote healing. *Br J Plast Surg* 1998; 51: 79.
7. Meguid MM, Debonis D, Meduid V, *et al.* Complications of abdominal operations for malignant disease. *Am J Surg* 1988; 156: 341-5.
8. Mughal MM, Meduid MM. The effect of nutritional status on morbidity after elective surgery for benign gastrointestinal disease. *JPEN J Parenter Enteral Nutr* 1987; 11: 140-3.
9. Gonzalez-Pinto I, Gonzalez EM. Optimising the treatment of upper gastrointestinal fistulae. *Gut* 2001; 49 (Suppl4): iv22-iv31.
10. Lloyd DAJ, Gabe SM, Windsor ACJ. Nutrition and management of enterocutaneous fistula. *Br J Surg* 2006; 93: 1045-55.
11. Li J, Ren J, Zhu W, *et al.* Management of enterocutaneous fistulas: 30-year clinical experience. *Chin Med J (Engl)* 2003; 116: 171-5.
12. Deitel M. Elemental diet and enterocutaneous fistula. *World J Surg* 1983; 7: 451-4.
13. Doig GS, Heighes PT, Simpson F. Early enteral nutrition reduces mortality in trauma patients requiring intensive care: a meta-analysis of randomized controlled trials. *Injury* 2011; 42: 50-6.
14. Nightingale J, Woodward JM and Small Bowel and Nutrition Committee of the British Society of Gastroenterology. Guidelines for management of patients with a short bowel. *Gut* 2006; 55 (Suppl 4): 1-12.
15. Nightingale JM, Walker ER, Burnham WR, *et al.* Octreotide (a somatostatin analogue) improves the quality of life in some patients with a short intestine. *Aliment Pharmacol Ther* 1989; 3: 367-73.
16. NubiolaP, Badia JM, Martinez-Rodenas F, *et al.* Treatment of 27 postoperative enterocutaneous fistulas with the long half-life somatostatin analogue SMS 201-995. *Ann Surg* 1989; 210: 56-8.
17. Schwartz DA, Wiersema MJ, Dudiak KM, *et al.* A comparison of endoscopic ultrasound, magnetic resonance imaging, and exam under anesthesia for evaluation of Crohn's perianal fistulas. *Gastroenterology* 2001; 121: 1064-72.
18. Martinez D, Zibari G, Aultman D, *et al.* The outcome of intestinal fistulae: the Louisiana State University Medical Center - Shreveport experience. *Am Surg* 1998; 64: 252-4.
19. Garden OJ, Dykes EH, Carter DC. Surgical and nutritional management of postoperative duodenal fistulas. *Dig Dis Sci* 1988; 33: 30-5.
20. Hollington P, Mawdsley J, Lim W, *et al.* An 11-year experience of enterocutaneous fistula. *Br J Surg* 2004; 91: 1646-51.
21. Haffejee AA. Surgical management of high output enterocutaneous fistulae: a 24-year experience. *Curr Opin Clin Nutr Metab Care* 2004; 7: 309-16.

22. Campos AC, Andrade DF, Campos GM, *et al.* A multivariate model to determine prognostic factors in gastrointestinal fistulas. *J Am Coll Surg* 1999; 188: 483-90.
23. Reber HA, Roberts C, Way LW, Dunphy JE. Management of external gastrointestinal fistulas. *Ann Surg* 1978; 188: 460-7.
24. Lynch AC, Delaney CP, Senagore AJ, *et al.* Clinical outcome and factors predictive of recurrence after enterocutaneous fistula surgery. *Ann Surg* 2004; 240: 825-31.
25. Hill GL. Operative strategy in the treatment of enterocutaneous fistulas. *World J Surg* 1983; 7: 495-501.
26. Jones JH, Lennard-Jones JE. Corticosteroids and corticotrophin in the treatment of Crohn's disease. *Gut* 1966; 7: 181-7.
27. Bernstein LH, Frank MS, Brandt LJ, Boley SJ. Healing of perineal Crohn's disease with metronidazole. *Gastroenterology* 1980; 79: 599.
28. West RL, Van Der Woude CJ, Hansen BE, *et al.* Clinical and endosonographic effect of ciprofloxacin on the treatment of perianal fistulae in Crohn's disease with infliximab: a double-blind placebo-controlled study. *Aliment Pharmacol Ther* 2004; 20(11-12): 1329-36.
29. Pearson DC, May GR, Fick GH, Sutherland LR. Azathioprine and 6-mercaptopurine in Crohn disease. A meta-analysis. *Ann Intern Med* 1995; 123: 132-42.
30. Egan LJ, Sandborn WJ, Tremaine WJ. Clinical outcome following treatment of refractory inflammatory and fistulizing Crohn's disease with intravenous cyclosporine. *Am J Gastroenterol* 1998; 93: 442-8.
31. Present DH, Lichtiger S. Efficacy of cyclosporine in treatment of fistula of Crohn's disease. *Digestive Dis Sci* 1994; 39: 374-80.
32. Sandborn WJ, Present DH, Isaacs KL, *et al.* Tacrolimus for the treatment of fistulas in patients with Crohn's disease: a randomized, placebo-controlled trial. *Gastroenterology* 2003; 125: 380-8.
33. Present DH, Rutgeerts P, Targan S *et al.* Infliximab for the treatment of fistulas in patients with Crohn's disease. *New Engl J Med* 1990; 340: 1398-405.
34. Sands BE, Anderson FH, Bernstein CN, *et al.* Infliximab maintenance therapy for fistulizing Crohn's disease. *New Engl J Med* 2004; 350: 876-85.
35. Colombel J-F, Sandborn WJ, Rutgeerts P, *et al.* Adalimumab for maintenance of clinical response and remission in patients with Crohn's disease: the CHARM trial. *Gastroenterology* 2007; 132: 52-65.
36. Schreiber S, Lawrance IC, Thomsen OØ, *et al.* Randomised clinical trial: certolizumab pegol for fistulas in Crohn's disease - subgroup results from a placebo-controlled study. *Aliment Pharmacol Ther* 2011; 33: 185-93.
37. Ochsenküh T, Göke B, Sackmann M. Combining infliximab with 6-mercaptopurine/azathioprine for fistula therapy in Crohn's disease. *Am J Gastroenterol* 2002; 97: 2022-5.
38. Sands BE, Blank MA, Patel K, *et al.* Long-term treatment of rectovaginal fistulas in Crohn's disease: response to infliximab in the ACCENT II study. *Clin Gastroenterol Hepatol* 2004; 2: 912-20.
39. Vavricka SR, Rogler G. Fistula treatment: the unresolved challenge. *Dig Dis* 2010; 28: 556-64.

Chapter 14

Oral and upper gastrointestinal Crohn's disease

Kirstin M. Taylor BSc MRCP Clinical Research Fellow, Guy's & St Thomas' NHS Foundation Trust & King's College London, UK
Helen Campbell BSc SRD Dietitian, Guy's & St Thomas' NHS Foundation Trust, London, UK
Jeremy Sanderson MD FRCP Consultant Gastroenterologist, Guy's & St. Thomas' NHS Foundation Trust; Reader in Gastroenterology, Department of Nutrition, King's College London, UK

Overview

Oral manifestations of Crohn's disease (CD) fall into two types: true oral CD and 'extraintestinal' oral manifestations. Oral CD is a disfiguring condition more commonly termed orofacial granulomatosis and less than 25% of patients have involvement elsewhere in the gastrointestinal tract. Dietary treatment is first-line therapy, although in some cases topical or systemic immunosuppression is required.

Upper gastrointestinal CD is an aggressive variant and requires early diagnosis and treatment. Proton pump inhibitors are important in the management of oesophageal and gastroduodenal CD, but severe disease may require treatment with systemic immunosuppressants and anti-TNF drugs. Nutrition and conservative surgery are key management strategies in jejunal disease.

Introduction

The Vienna classification (1998) defined upper gastrointestinal (UGI) Crohn's disease (CD) as "any disease proximal to the terminal ileum (excluding the oral cavity) with or without additional involvement of the terminal ileum or colon" [1]. This potentially grouped together patients with either proximal disease alone or both proximal and distal disease. The Montreal classification therefore revised this definition so that UGI CD was added as a separate and additional site to distal disease [2]. The separation of oral CD is important because this does appear to be a somewhat unique entity requiring quite specific management approaches. Hence, we have divided this chapter into two parts. In each we discuss the presentation and management of these often challenging aspects of CD.

Presentation and management of oral Crohn's disease

Definition and nomenclature

The oral manifestations of CD fall into two types: the first is true oral CD, entirely distinct from the second, which is the 'extraintestinal' oral manifestation. Extraintestinal oral manifestations include recurrent aphthous ulceration, often occurring as crops of painful aphthous ulcers at times of flare-ups of intestinal CD and are sometimes associated with nutritional deficit (vitamin B12, folate, iron). The extraintestinal type also includes glossitis, angular cheilitis (both often also linked to haematinic deficiency) and oral candidiasis (particularly in those on corticosteroids). It is also of note that dentition in patients with severe CD can be affected as a consequence of malnutrition and cumulative steroid exposure.

True oral CD is best included under the umbrella term of orofacial granulomatosis (OFG), a disfiguring condition which covers all granulomatous diseases affecting the oral cavity and perioral facial skin, other examples of which might include tuberculosis, sarcoidosis and the Melkersson Rosenthal syndrome (MRS) [3]. OFG is rare though the true incidence and aetiology are unknown. Currently no epidemiological studies exist although the majority of publications are from the UK and patient numbers would seem comparatively higher in the West of

Scotland [4]. Most patients with OFG are young and present with only oral manifestations. Less than one-quarter also have a concurrent diagnosis of gastrointestinal CD [5]. Sarcoidosis and tuberculosis are rarely seen as the primary cause of this disease [6]. MRS is very rarely seen and is suggested by concurrent facial palsy and fissuring of the tongue. A proportion of cases of OFG (approximately 64%) can present with microscopic and macroscopic gastrointestinal changes on colonoscopy but otherwise remain relatively asymptomatic requiring no intervention for gastrointestinal management [7]. Diagnosis is made on oral examination and confirmed by oral biopsy. The histological findings include deep-seated non-caseating epithelioid granulomas and multinucleated Langhans type giant cells within the oral mucosa [8]. Negative biopsies, however, should not exclude a diagnosis of OFG as the clinical findings are quite characteristic.

Clinical presentation

Chronic lip swelling (Figure 1) is the most common presentation and the one which patients find most distressing contributing substantially to

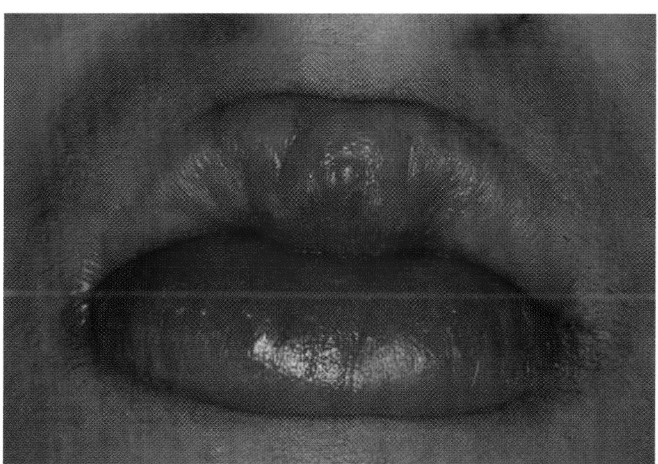

Figure 1. Orofacial granulomatosis. Erythema and swelling of upper and lower lips with angular cheilitis.

the disproportionate psychological morbidity seen in this condition. Facial swelling and erythema, often spreading from the lips, can occur, increasing the facial disfigurement. Intra-orally, patients may also present with nodular buccal swelling, sometimes termed buccal cobblestoning, similar to that seen in the intestine in CD [5]. Florid pink gingivae might be indicative of granulomatous inflammation. Less commonly, in the floor of the mouth, swelling of the sublingual and submandibular salivary duct orifices is seen, known as 'staghorning' and is highly characteristic of OFG. The tongue, palate (soft and hard), and oropharynx are only rarely involved. Linear oral ulceration may be present, especially in the buccal sulcus, a finding that might be indicative of concurrent gastrointestinal CD. Abnormal blood tests including anaemia, and raised inflammatory parameters are suggestive of concurrent intestinal CD and hence might help to indicate patients in whom gut investigation should be undertaken. Angular cheilitis and other lip fissures require routine swabs for microscopy and culture because, where present, treatment of superimposed candida or bacterial infections can help reduce associated inflammation.

The majority of patients with gastrointestinal CD do not develop oral CD. In patients with oral involvement alone, the likelihood of developing gut CD is not known but there is evidence that childhood onset might be a more predisposing trait. Overall, however, the risk is thought to be relatively low. The implications are that gastrointestinal investigation is not necessary in all patients with OFG and should only be carried out in patients with gastrointestinal symptoms. Similarly, a small proportion of patients can present with perianal (or genital) involvement, so called oroanal and orogenital granulomatosis, for which no other gastrointestinal involvement or symptoms are apparent. Again, gut investigations in such individuals need only be carried out if there are other signs suggestive of a diagnosis of gut CD [5].

Management

The long-term management of OFG can be difficult and sometimes disappointing. No structured treatment protocols exist but the primary treatment (irrespective of a concurrent diagnosis of CD) includes a cinnamon and benzoate-free diet [5]. The mechanism of action is unclear but benefit can be seen in up to three-quarters of patients [9]. Other dietary treatments include a liquid enteral diet and, in particular, an elemental diet has proven to be successful particularly in childhood disease [10]. After diet, other treatments are similar to that of CD and usually involve immunomodulatory therapy such as thiopurines [11] and anti-TNF therapy in refractory OFG [12]. Oral corticosteroids are reserved for significant flare-ups, as in CD elsewhere in the gastrointestinal tract, and intralesional steroid injections can be used, particularly for the acute management of significant lip involvement. Less invasive measures for mild disease include beclomethasone mouthwashes and topical tacrolimus ointment. Other less common but reportedly beneficial treatments have included clofazamine [8] and thalidomide [13], but the latter has significant limitations, not just for use in women of childbearing age but also because of drowsiness and peripheral neuropathy. In the event of long-term severe disfiguring fibrotic lip disease, debulking cheilopasty might be necessary, somewhat akin to the resection of fibrotic strictures in gut CD [6].

Upper gastrointestinal Crohn's disease

Upper gastrointestinal Crohn's disease (UGI CD) is rare in adult patients with CD, with a prevalence rate between less than 1% and 10% (see Table 1) [14]. This proportion of patients with UGI CD is higher if radiological, endoscopic and histological findings are taken into account;

Table 1. Prevalence of UGI Crohn's disease in adults.

Site	Prevalence [14]
Oesophageal	<1%
Gastric	<1%
Duodenal	2-10%
Jejunal/jejuno-ileal	3-10%

however, only clinically significant disease is relevant when considering therapy. In children, UGI CD is more prevalent, with up to 36% affected at diagnosis, increasing to as high as 48% at longer-term follow-up [15]. It is recommended that children with suspected CD are initially investigated with both ileocolonoscopy and UGI endoscopy, as well as small bowel imaging [16]. UGI endoscopy is not recommended as part of the initial investigation in adults with suspected CD unless patients have UGI symptoms.

Genetically, *NOD2* variants and association with CD, in particular ileal involvement, stricturing behaviour and younger age at diagnosis, are well described. Patients with gastroduodenal CD have been found to be more likely than those with distal disease alone to have two of the three major allelic *NOD2* variants (*G908R*, *L1007P* and *R702W*) and to be homozygous for *L1007P* [17].

There is a lack of controlled trials of therapy in UGI CD, despite the fact that more proximal disease is associated with a poorer prognosis. The majority of evidence-based therapy is derived from case series. Patients are often already on immunosuppressant therapy for co-existing distal disease.

Oesophageal Crohn's disease

The typical presentation of oesophageal CD is with dysphagia, but odynophagia, heartburn, chest pain may also be presenting symptoms. The diagnosis is usually made at UGI endoscopy, with erythema, erosions, ulceration both superficial and deep (Figure 2), and stricturing. No one site of strictures in the oesophagus predominates. Fistulae are very rare and if present usually communicate with the bronchial tree. The histology is often non-specific with characteristic granulomas and giant cells present in less than 25 of cases.

Acid-suppressing therapies, such as proton pump inhibitors, can help with oesophageal symptoms [18]. Topical corticosteroids can be used and in particular ingestion of an aerosolised steroid, such as budesonide, has had some success [19]. Severe disease may require treatment with anti-TNF therapy.

Strictures usually require serial balloon dilatations in conjunction with intra-lesional corticosteroid injections. Topical post-dilatation application of mitomycin-C (an antiproliferative agent that inhibits fibroblast proliferation and activity) can reduce both symptomatic and endoscopic recurrence [20]. Oesophagectomy may be required in patients with disease refractory to medical and endoscopic therapy. Stents have been used, and the advent of biodegradable stents may offer a treatment approach helping to prevent surgery.

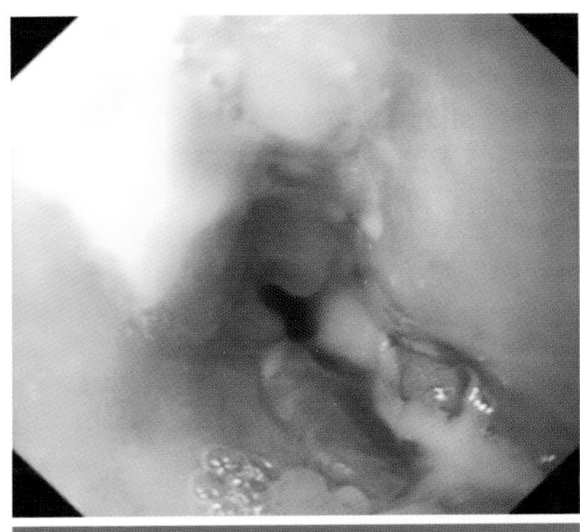

Figure 2. Endoscopic view of oesophageal Crohn's disease.

Gastroduodenal Crohn's disease

The symptoms of gastroduodenal CD are varied but include epigastric pain, nausea, vomiting, early satiety, anorexia, bloating and weight loss. Symptoms related to duodenal involvement with a component of gastric outlet obstruction are the commonest presentation.

True involvement of the stomach is rare. Three-quarters of patients with distal CD have a *Helicobacter pylori*-negative gastritis on biopsy [21]. Contiguous inflammation involving the antrum, pylorus and proximal duodenum is the most common pattern of disease. Endoscopic findings include erythema, erosions, lack of distensibility of the stomach, thickened gastric folds, cobblestoning, ulceration (both aphthous and serpiginous), notching of Kerkring's folds, and stricturing.

Acid suppression with a proton pump inhibitor is advocated, along with testing for and treatment of *H. pylori.* Aminosalicyates are generally not beneficial in UGI CD and may exacerbate symptoms. Drug treatment of active gastroduodenal inflammation is otherwise as for CD elsewhere, primarily with thiopurines and, where necessary, anti-TNF therapy [22]. Short pyloric and duodenal strictures can be balloon-dilated although this is often difficult and requires repeated attempts. One-third of patients are refractory to medical and endoscopic therapy and require surgery; most commonly gastrojejunostomy but additionally gastroduodenostomy, duodenojejunostomy or strictureplasty can be performed [23]. Fistulae in the stomach or duodenum are usually of ileal or colonic origin [14] and surgery is the treatment of choice.

Pancreatitis is a rare complication of CD and may arise due to ampullary stenosis/obstruction secondary to duodenal inflammation, or backwash of duodenal contents into the pancreatic duct. Duodenal adenocarcinoma on a background of longstanding duodenal CD has been reported but is exceptionally rare.

Jejunal Crohn's disease

Patients with jejunal involvement of CD may present with abdominal pain and cramps in the central or left upper quadrant of the abdomen relatively soon after eating. Nutritional deficit with associated weight loss and fatigue are particular problems in jejunal CD. In children this is reflected by growth retardation.

Patients with jejunal CD are younger at the time of development of symptoms, diagnosis and first operation than those with distal disease alone [24]. Endoscopic diagnosis is difficult as the inflammatory lesions are beyond the reach of standard UGI endoscopy and ileocolonoscopy. However, small bowel MRI (Figure 3)(enterography or enteroclysis) and ultrasound in experienced hands provide a non-invasive, reliable method of diagnosis and assessment of proximal disease, without resort to the

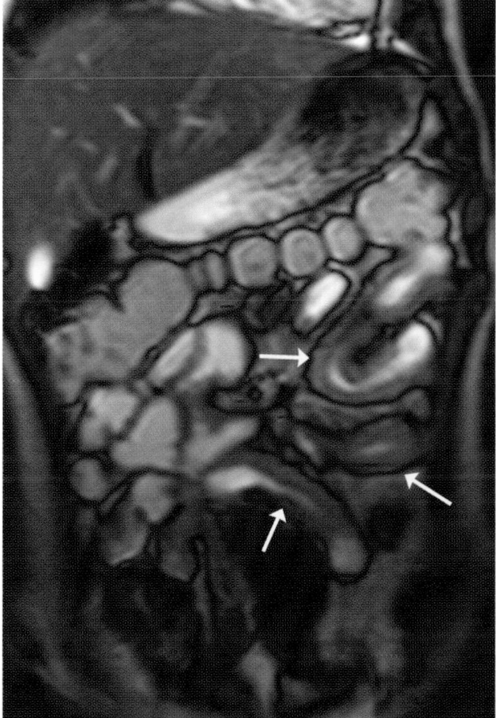

Figure 3. Jejunal Crohn's disease. Coronal true FISP MRI in a 14-year-old male patient with active jejunal Crohn's disease. There are multiple thick-walled loops of jejunum (arrows) separated by fibrofatty proliferation within the mesentery. *Courtesy of Dr Nyree Griffin.*

ionizing radiation required for small bowel barium studies. Wireless capsule endoscopy should be avoided in those in whom strictures are suspected, but gives good mucosal images of the whole small bowel and can identify more subtle disease not seen on imaging. Enteroscopy (push, spiral, single and double balloon) is more laborious and invasive but permits biopsies for histological analysis, and permits endoscopic therapy, particularly balloon dilatation, where indicated.

In view of the aggressive nature of jejunal CD, patients should be treated early with immunosuppression, including anti-TNF therapy, in order to preserve functioning small bowel length and to keep cumulative steroid dose as low as possible. Nutritional therapy (elemental or polymeric diets) can be used as primary therapy in those with milder disease but should also be considered as an adjunct in those requiring other treatments. In children this helps restore growth, independent of nutritional benefits.

In extensive disease, surgical resection risks the development of short bowel syndrome. Strictureplasty preserves bowel length and has comparable recurrence rates with resection. Jejunal CD is associated with a higher early postoperative recurrence than distal ileal disease and therefore the use of anti-TNF therapy and immunosuppression following surgery should be considered.

While stricturing is more common in jejunal CD than distal ileal disease, fistulisation appears to be rarer (10% vs. 34%), and does not depend on the presence of strictures [25]. Fistulae invariably require surgical resection, and often require a period of parenteral nutrition (PN). With improvements in medical therapy, nutritional support and conservative surgery, short bowel syndrome and intestinal failure are rare occurrences in CD. Hence, permanent parenteral nutrition and small bowel transplantation, whilst still options, are only rarely needed. For further details on jejunal Crohn's disease see Chapter 8.

Conclusions

Oral CD is a disfiguring condition more commonly termed orofacial granulomatosis, particularly in patients where no evidence of gastrointestinal involvement elsewhere is apparent. This challenging disease typically presents with chronic lip swelling in young adults and gastrointestinal involvement is seen in less than a quarter of patients. Dietary treatment is first-line therapy, and in some cases combination with topical immunosuppression is required. In refractory OFG, systemic immunosuppression is indicated.

UGI CD is an aggressive variant and requires early diagnosis and treatment. Advances in endoscopic techniques and imaging in the last decade allow accurate assessment of parts of the bowel that were previously difficult to reach. Assessment of the proximal gut at diagnosis is important, particularly in children, even when more distal disease is present. The principles of management vary according to the site involved. Jejunal CD is challenging to treat; nutritional therapy and conservative surgery are the key management strategies.

Key points

- **Oral manifestations of CD are common but true oral Crohn's is rare.**
- **True oral Crohn's has some unique management aspects, particularly dietary treatment, and should be assessed and managed in a specialist centre, with the input of oral surgeons, gastroenterologists and dietitians.**
- **In children, UGI assessment should be undertaken at initial investigation.**
- **In adults, there should be a low threshold for initiation of UGI investigations for those in whom UGI CD is suspected.**
- **UGI CD is often a herald of a more aggressive disease course and therefore early treatment with immunosuppression and biological therapy should be considered.**

References

1. Gasche C, Scholmerich J, Brynskov J, *et al.* A simple classification of Crohn's disease: report of the Working Party for the World Congresses of Gastroenterology, Vienna 1998. *Inflamm Bowel Dis* 2000; 6: 8-15.
2. Silverberg MS, Satsangi J, Ahmad T, *et al.* Toward an integrated clinical, molecular and serological classification of inflammatory bowel disease: Report of a Working Party of the 2005 Montreal World Congress of Gastroenterology. *Canadian Journal of Gastroenterology* 2005; 19 Suppl A: 5-36.

3. Wiesenfeld D, Ferguson MM, Mitchell DN, *et al.* Oro-facial granulomatosis - a clinical and pathological analysis. *Q J Med* 1985; 54(213): 101-13.
4. Gibson J, Wray D, Bagg J. Oral staphylococcal mucositis: a new clinical entity in orofacial granulomatosis and Crohn's disease. *Oral Surg Oral Med Oral Pathol Oral Radiol Endod* 2000; 89: 171-6.
5. Campbell H, Escudier M, Patel P, *et al.* Distinguishing orofacial granulomatosis from Crohn's disease: two separate disease entities? *Inflamm Bowel Dis* 2011; 17: 2109-15
6. Grave B, McCullough M, Wiesenfeld D. Orofacial granulomatosis - a 20-year review. *Oral Dis* 2009; 15: 46-51.
7. Sanderson J, Nunes C, Escudier M, *et al.* Oro-facial granulomatosis: Crohn's disease or a new inflammatory bowel disease? *Inflamm Bowel Dis* 2005; 11: 840-6.
8. van der Waal RI, Schulten EA, van der Meij EH, *et al.* Cheilitis granulomatosa: overview of 13 patients with long-term follow-up - results of management. *Int J Dermatol* 2002; 41: 225-9.
9. White A, Nunes C, Escudier M, *et al.* Improvement in orofacial granulomatosis on a cinnamon- and benzoate-free diet. *Inflamm Bowel Dis* 2006; 12: 508-14.
10. Kiparissi F, Lindley K, Hill S, *et al.* Orofacial granulomatosis is a separate entity of Crohn's disease comprising an allergic component. *Journal of Pediatric Gastroenterology and Nutriton* 2006; 42: E3.
11. Plauth M, Jenss H, Meyle J. Oral manifestations of Crohn's disease. An analysis of 79 cases. *J Clin Gastroenterol* 1991; 13: 29-37.
12. Elliott E, Campbell H, Escudier M, *et al.* Experience with anti-TNF-alpha therapy for orofacial granulomatosis. *J Oral Pathol Med* 2011; 40: 14-9.
13. Hegarty A, Hodgson T, Porter S. Thalidomide for the treatment of recalcitrant oral Crohn's disease and orofacial granulomatosis. *Oral Surg Oral Med Oral Pathol Oral Radiol Endod* 2003; 95: 576-85.
14. van Hogezand RA, Witte AM, Veenendaal RA, *et al.* Proximal Crohn's disease: review of the clinicopathologic features and therapy. *Inflamm Bowel Dis* 2001; 7: 328-37.
15. Vernier-Massouille G, Balde M, Salleron J, *et al.* Natural history of pediatric Crohn's disease: a population-based cohort study. *Gastroenterology* 2008; 135: 1106-13.
16. Escher JC, Amil Dias J, Bochenek K. Inflammatory bowel disease in children and adolescents. Recommendations for diagnosis: the Porto criteria. Medical position paper: IBD working group of the European Society for Paediatric Gastroenterology, Hepatology and Nutrition (ESPGHAN). *Journal of Pediatric Gastroenterology and Nutriton* 2005; 41: 1-7.
17. Mardini HE, Gregory KJ, Nasser M, *et al.* Gastroduodenal Crohn's disease is associated with *NOD2/CARD15* gene polymorphisms, particularly *L1007P* homozygosity. *Dig Dis Sci* 2005; 50(12): 2316-22.
18. Decker GAG, Loftus EV, Pasha TM, *et al.* Crohn's disease of the esophagus: clinical features and outcomes. *Inflamm Bowel Dis* 2001; 7: 113-9.
19. Zezos P, Kouklakis G, Oikonomou A, *et al.* Esophageal Crohn's disease treated 'topically' with swallowed aerosolized budesonide. *Case Report Med* pii: 418769. Epub 2010 Sep 30.

20. Rosseneu S, Afzal N, Yerushalmi B, *et al.* Topical application of mitomycin-C in oesophageal strictures. *J Pediatr Gastroenterol Nutr* 2007; 44: 336-41.
21. Oberhuber G, Puspok A, Oesterreicher C, *et al.* Focally enhanced gastritis: a frequent type of gastritis in patients with Crohn's disease. *Gastroenterology* 1997; 112: 698-706.
22. Knapp AB, Mirsky FJ, Dillon EH, Korelitz BI. Successful infliximab therapy for a duodenal stricture caused by Crohn's disease. *Inflamm Bowel Dis* 2005; 11: 1123-5.
23. Marcello PW, Schoetz DJ Jr. Gastroduodenal Crohn's disease: surgical management. In: *Advanced Therapy of Inflammatory Bowel Disease*. Bayless TM, Hanauer SB, Eds. Hamilton, Ontario: BC Decker, 2001: 461-3.
24. Munkholm P, Langholz E, Davidsen M, Binder V. Disease activity courses in a regional cohort of Crohn's disease patients. *Scand J Gastroenterol* 1995; 30: 699-706.
25. Marion JF, Lachman P, Greenstein AJ, Sachar DB. Rarity of fistulas in Crohn's disease of the jejunum. *Inflamm Bowel Dis* 1995; 1: 34-6.

Part 3 Introduction

Current issues in other scenarios

Ailsa L. Hart BMBCh MRCP PhD Senior Clinical Lecturer, Imperial College and Consultant Gastroenterologist, St Mark's Hospital, London, UK

Patients with IBD have many health issues not only related to their gastrointestinal tracts but also extraintestinal manifestations (Chapter 15), such as skin lesions (erythema nodosum, pyoderma gangrenosum), eye symptoms (uveitis, episcleritis), joint pains (peripheral arthritis, ankylosing spondylitis, sacroiliitis) and liver involvement (primary sclerosing cholangitis).

Patients with longstanding ulcerative colitis and Crohn's colitis have an increased risk of colorectal cancer and surveillance colonoscopies are recommended (Chapter 16). Those with longstanding, extensive ulcerative colitis or colonic Crohn's disease are approximately six times more likely to develop colorectal cancer than the general population. Recently there has been an improved understanding of the risk factors associated with colorectal cancer development and the natural history of dysplasia in patients with IBD. New endoscopic techniques have been developed to enhance surveillance and the British Society of

Gastroenterology (BSG) recommends surveillance colonoscopies yearly, 3-yearly or 5-yearly depending on the risk factors.

Many patients with IBD are of childbearing age and ask questions about fertility, pregnancy and breastfeeding. A careful discussion of effects of active disease on pregnancy outcome as well as side effects of medications used to treat active disease is needed with a multidisciplinary approach between the gastroenterologist, surgeon and obstetrician (Chapter 17).

Opportunistic infections have emerged as an important safety issue in patients with IBD, especially with increasing use of immunomodulator therapy and biologics. Gastroenterologists need to recognise, prevent and treat common and uncommon infections (Chapter 18).

Management of adolescents with IBD is in many ways similar to treating adults with IBD, but special consideration needs to be given to the impact on growth of both the disease and the therapies used, and to their individual psychosocial needs (Chapter 19).

Anaemia is common in patients with IBD with iron deficiency and anaemia of chronic disease being the main causes. Optimum treatment of anaemia in IBD includes controlling inflammation, replenishing deficient micronutrients, and ensuring adequate nutrition (Chapter 20).

IBD is associated with bone diseases including osteoporosis, osteopenia and vitamin D deficiency, which need to be prevented and treated (Chapter 21).

Chapter 15

Extraintestinal manifestations of inflammatory bowel disease

Timothy R. Orchard MA MD DM FHEA FRCP Consultant Gastroenterologist, Imperial College Healthcare Trust and Reader in Gastroenterology, Imperial College London, St Mary's Hospital, London, UK

Evangelos A. Russo MBBS MRCP Clinical Research Fellow and Honorary Specialist Registrar in Gastroenterology, Imperial College London, Clinical Imaging Centre, Hammersmith Hospital, London, UK

Overview

Extraintestinal manifestations (EIMs) are a common occurrence in IBD patients, involving particularly the skin, the axial and peripheral locomotor systems, the eyes and the biliary tree. Epidemiological and genome-wide association studies have identified populations who are particularly high risk for one or more of these manifestations. Common cutaneous manifestations include erythema nodosum and pyoderma gangrenosum, whereas musculoskeletal complaints include axial arthritis as well as two distinct types of peripheral joint involvement which can sometimes co-exist with the spondylitis. Ocular manifestations vary from the relatively minor episcleritis to more serious sight-threatening inflammation of deeper layers, so a low threshold for specialist referral is advocated. Finally, primary sclerosing cholangitis is also a common EIM affecting the biliary tree, frequently progressing to cirrhosis and liver failure. Independently to their effect on the underlying disease, novel anti-TNFα medications have had an impact in the control of several of the extraintestinal symptoms.

Introduction

Patients with inflammatory bowel disease (IBD) frequently exhibit a variety of systemic complications collectively termed extraintestinal manifestations (EIMs), which contribute significantly to the condition's morbidity and effect on quality of life. Recent reports in the published literature estimate the prevalence of EIMs at 40% of IBD patients [1], and the majority of the organ systems may be affected.

Epidemiological studies suggest that being of African-American or Hispanic origin [2] is a possible risk factor in the development of at least a subset of EIMs and more recently, several gene associations in addition to the long-established HLA-B27 genotype have been proposed. The majority of EIMs, however, are still linked to IBD through epidemiological research rather than robustly established pathogenic pathways. The most widely proposed mechanism to date is that of one or more auto-antigens shared between the gut and the major extraintestinal organs [3]. The aim of this review is to examine the clinical presentation, pathogenesis and up-to-date management of the most frequently encountered EIMs of IBD.

Cutaneous manifestations

Erythema nodosum

Erythema nodosum (EN) is the commonest cutaneous manifestation of IBD. Its prevalence is reported to be between 5 and 10%, whereas some studies estimate it as high as 15% [4]. Women are more commonly affected than men and it is more prevalent in Crohn's disease [4]. EN lesions are typically found in the pre-tibial areas although the thighs and extensor aspects of forearms are also occasionally involved. Their characteristic macroscopic appearance is that of raised, warm, tender nodules whilst histological assessment typically reveals septal panniculitis secondary to immune complex deposition [5].

EN lesions associated with IBD are frequently recurrent, and flares typically occur concurrently with intestinal exacerbations [4].

Pain and swelling from EN lesions generally resolve spontaneously within 3-6 weeks, whereas the associated discolouration may persist for a few months. Supportive management is largely non-evidence-based and includes non-steroidal anti-inflammatory drugs (NSAIDs), potassium iodide, bed rest and compression-elevation of the affected limb. However, NSAIDs should be used with caution, as they may cause relapse of IBD [6]. In difficult cases the skin lesions themselves may require systemic corticosteroid therapy, and on occasion even immunomodulators. However, in general, treatment of the underlying gut disease is the most effective strategy and leads to resolution of the EN [7].

Pyoderma gangrenosum

Pyoderma gangrenosum (PG) occurs less frequently than EN, with an estimated prevalence of up to 2%. It can occur anywhere in the body but most commonly involves the shins as well as areas around surgical stomata. Macroscopically, PG is described as discrete pustules during the initial phases of its natural history, which then coalesce and form ulcerations with erythematous or violaceous edges. Histological analysis reveals a deep suppurative folliculitis with dense neutrophilic and lymphocytic infiltrate [8].

In contrast to EN, pyoderma frequently runs a course independent of the underlying inflammation. Specific therapy for PG can be either topical or systemic. The former involves the principles of moist wound management with foam or laminate dressings or, in the case of excess slough or suppuration, saline-soaked compresses. In addition, the successful use of topical corticosteroids, 5-ASAs and calcineurin inhibitors has been reported.

High-dose corticosteroids, with or without minocycline, is a sensible first-line systemic option supported by Level B evidence. In more severe cases, pulsed methylprednisolone of 1g daily over 3-5 days has also been tried with some success [9]. Frequently, however, steroids are ineffective or undesirable, and other therapies are required. The evidence base is poor for most treatments, but first-line immune suppression for PG is normally with a calcineurin inhibitor such as cyclosporine or tacrolimus. For small patches of PG, topical tacrolimus paste has been used with some success in small series. There is more robust evidence for the use of infliximab, which was given in a trial setting and showed efficacy; however, it was given as a single dose, and the PG often recurred. There is no evidence about longer-term therapy, and combination with an immune suppressant such as azathioprine may be a sensible approach [10-12].

Musculoskeletal manifestations

Musculoskeletal manifestations are the commonest EIMs associated with IBD and are considered to be part of a wider group termed seronegative spondyloarthropathies. They are subdivided into axial disease, affecting up to 6% of patients, with asymptomatic sacro-iliitis being a far commoner *form fruste*, and peripheral arthritis. The latter, affecting 5-20% of IBD sufferers, is further subdivided into Type 1, a pauci-articular large joint arthritis typically running a parallel course to the intestinal illness, and Type 2, a symmetric small joint poly-arthropathy that flares independently from the gut [13].

Axial disease

IBD-associated ankylosing spondylitis

IBD-associated ankylosing spondylitis (AS) has similar clinical and radiological features as idiopathic AS, characterised by inflammatory back pain and radiological changes. Around 30% of patients also have objective peripheral locomotor involvement in addition to the axial disease. Unlike idiopathic AS the male:female ratio in IBD-associated AS is roughly 1:1 (i.e. no male preponderance). Interestingly, the HLA-B27 association seen in idiopathic AS is also found in IBD-AS but it is much weaker (5-70% vs. 94%) [14, 15]. Other genetic associations with AS have been described which may account for some of this difference, but much of it is likely to relate to the presence of gut inflammation, suggesting that the gut has an important role in its aetiology [16].

Isolated sacro-iliitis

Whilst AS is a well-defined clinical syndrome characterised by the presence of inflammatory low back pain associated with radiological changes of sacro-iliitis on MRI or plain radiology, a large number of IBD patients may present with changes of sacro-iliitis on imaging, but with little in the way of symptoms. The numbers involved vary depending on the imaging modality used but may be up to 20% using plain radiology and 40% using MRI scanning. The correct approach to management is unknown. A pragmatic approach is to conduct a full rheumatological history and examination including measurements of lumbar spinal flexion, and to test for HLA-B27. If patients are symptomatic, have decreased range of movements or are HLA-B27-positive, they should be referred for a rheumatological opinion and possible physical therapy in the first instance, and may require more intervention. If they are asymptomatic with a normal range of movements and HLA-B27-negative, a conservative approach may be taken, monitoring the spine at intervals.

Peripheral arthropathies

IBD-related peripheral arthropathies are commoner in females and occasionally pre-date the onset of the intestinal symptoms. They are distinguished by the fact that they are not erosive or deforming in the way that psoriatic or rheumatoid arthritis are, but they may be persistent or recurrent and can give rise to significant morbidity.

Type 1 arthritis typically presents as a migratory non-deforming and non-erosive large-joint arthropathy involving less than five joints which clinically demonstrate swelling and/or effusion. It is less strongly linked with HLA-B27 than axial disease, and more specific genotypic associations are with HLA-B35 and, in particular, HLA-DRB1-0103 present in up to 65% of patients versus 3% of controls [17]. Its natural history is that of an acute self-limiting episode lasting up to 10 weeks which is typically associated with an IBD flare.

Features of Type 2 arthritis on the other hand are those of a persistent symmetrical non-deforming poly-arthropathy that runs an independent course to the underlying bowel disease, frequently persisting well beyond gut symptom resolution [18]. The only known specific genetic association is with HLA-B44 possessed by 62% of patients.

Current therapeutics of IBD-related AS and peripheral arthritis

Treatment of IBD-AS is identical to that of idiopathic AS, and should be conducted in collaboration with a rheumatologist. Physical therapies are vital in preventing deformity and loss of range of movement. Non-steroidals may be used with caution, as they may cause relapse of IBD even in quiescent disease [6]. Methotrexate may be used for associated peripheral disease, but is not effective for axial disease. Anti-TNF therapy is effective for symptoms of axial disease, but there is controversy over whether it affects long-term progression. If an anti-TNF agent is required in IBD-AS, it is probably sensible to use infliximab or adalimumab (which have been shown to be effective in IBD) rather than etanercept.

As the peripheral arthropathies of IBD are not deforming or erosive, treatment is generally aimed at symptomatic relief, and in the first instance this means simple analgesia. NSAIDs may be tried in quiescent disease but may induce a flare in up to 28% of patients even from a quiescent state [6], and so must be used with caution. Compound analgesics may produce constipation which is unwelcome, especially by people with distal colitis, but may be a safer option.

If the gut disease is active then treatment of the underlying gut inflammation is often effective in relieving the joint problems. If specific treatment is required, sulfasalazine and even mesalazine have shown some modest symptomatic benefits [19]. When escalation beyond these therapies is deemed necessary there is little evidence to support specific treatments, but systemic corticosteroids, azathioprine or methotrexate have all been used in these patients. The advent of anti-TNFα agents, however, has significantly improved outcomes in this cohort of peripheral disease in small case series [20-22].

Ocular manifestations

Clinical presentations

Symptomatic ocular manifestations occur in between 3-12% of IBD patients, whereas up to 43% of patients were found to have positive examination findings on routine screening in one study [23]. There is a well-documented clustering of ocular and locomotor EIMs in the same patients [3]. Most anatomical compartments of the eye may be involved, producing sequelae of variable severity.

Superficially, episcleritis is the commonest ocular manifestation, typically flaring and subsiding at the same time as the gut [24]. It presents with ocular irritation and superficial erythema with or without pain. Visual acuity and pupillary reflexes are characteristically preserved. Scleritis on the contrary produces more severe pain, profound purple discolouration and may threaten sight through retinal detachment or optic nerve oedema and as such it requires urgent ophthalmologic referral.

Inflammation of the deep vascular coat of the eye, i.e the iris, ciliary body and choroid is collectively termed uveitis, with the anterior chamber structures being more commonly involved in IBD patients. HLA-B27, B58, and HLA-DRB10103 genotypes confer a higher risk [4]. Episodes can run an independent course to the underlying bowel disease. Patients present with pain, photophobia and often profound visual loss. Clinically a characteristic redness that radiates out from the limbus can be observed while papillary responses are often abnormal.

Current therapeutics in IBD-related ocular disease

Episcleritis usually responds to conservative management with cold compresses occasionally requiring topical steroid preparations and it has an excellent prognosis.

In the case of suspected deeper inflammation, either of the sclera or the uvea, the importance of prompt specialist referral cannot be over-emphasised. Topical (inc. intra-ocular) or systemic corticosteroids is the preferred initial therapeutic approach. In cases of intolerance, lack of efficacy or conditions necessitating prolonged therapy, a plethora of immunomodulatory agents are also employed. There has been grade B evidence recommending the use of most immunomodulators currently in use for intestinal inflammation, in the treatment of ocular inflammatory disease, including methotrexate, azathioprine, and calcineurin inhibitors [25].

As is the case with the majority of EIMs, biologic therapies have also gained a role in the field of ocular inflammation. The main body of the evidence, however, still consists of retrospective case series and small pilot studies, or is extrapolated from cohorts of patients with ocular inflammatory disease of a wide aetiology [26-29].

Primary sclerosing cholangitis

Primary sclerosing cholangitis (PSC) is a chronic, slowly progressive cholestatic liver disease eventually leading to cirrhosis and liver failure. Up to 4% of patients with UC develop PSC [30], which can also be non-IBD-related in 30% of cases.

Whilst the majority of patients are identified at the asymptomatic phase, common symptoms include fatigue, generalised pruritus, jaundice and fever [31].

The mainstay of management of PSC over the last decades has been with ursodeoxycholic acid (UDCA), one of the hydrophilic bile acids. Suggested mechanisms of action are stabilisation of cell membranes, competitive inhibition of toxic bile acid absorption at the terminal ileum and a potential immunomodulatory effect. A recent Cochrane review of eight randomised, placebo-controlled trials on the use of UDCA in PSC disappointingly showed that despite a good safety and tolerability profile as well as efficacy in liver function test improvement, it failed to reach significance in hard endpoints such as death prevention, treatment failure (defined as the need for liver transplantation or hepatic decompensation), and histologic deterioration [32].

Evidence on conventional immunosuppression with steroids and anti-metabolites has been weak and results inconsistent. Some encouraging reports on regimes combining UDCA with steroids and immunomodulation suggest that larger-scale studies in this approach may be warranted [30]. The only prospective placebo-controlled trial on anti-TNFα therapy in PSC was terminated early because of clear lack of efficacy [33].

There is also a role for endoscopic management in PSC, through dilatation of dominant strictures, whereas, ultimately, liver transplantation is frequently necessary for such patients.

Conclusions

Extraintestinal manifestations are a significant burden for patients with inflammatory bowel disease. Prompt recognition and targeted therapy is vital in the management of such patients. The recent advent of biologic therapies has markedly improved clinical outcomes, through better control of the intestinal disease as well as potent anti-inflammatory effects at extraintestinal foci.

Key points

- **Extraintestinal manifestations (EIMs) of inflammatory bowel disease (IBD) are relatively common and may be associated with active IBD (large joint arthritis, erythema nodosum [EN], eye manifestations) or run a course independent of IBD (primary sclerosing cholangitis [PSC], ankylosing spondylitis [AS], small joint arthritis).**
- **There is probably a genetic predisposition to developing mucocutaneous EIMs related to the HLA complex.**
- **Therapy is aimed at treating symptoms, controlling underlying gut inflammation and specific therapy of the EIM.**
- **If specific therapy is required, systemic steroids, calcineurin inhibitors and anti-TNF strategies may be used.**
- **In severe or persistent cases specialist opinion should be sought, particularly in relation to eye disease.**

References

1. Ricart E, Panaccione R, Loftus EV, Jr., *et al.* Autoimmune disorders and extraintestinal manifestations in first-degree familial and sporadic inflammatory bowel disease: a case-control study. *Inflamm Bowel Dis* 2004; 10: 207-14.
2. Hou JK, El-Serag H, Thirumurthi S. Distribution and manifestations of inflammatory bowel disease in Asians, Hispanics, and African Americans: a systematic review. *Am J Gastroenterol* 2009; 104: 2100-9.
3. Das KM. Relationship of extraintestinal involvements in inflammatory bowel disease: new insights into autoimmune pathogenesis. *Dig Dis Sci* 1999; 44: 1-13.
4. Orchard TR, Chua CN, Ahmad T, *et al.* Uveitis and erythema nodosum in inflammatory bowel disease: clinical features and the role of HLA genes. *Gastroenterology* 2002; 123: 714-8.
5. Gilchrist H, Patterson JW. Erythema nodosum and erythema induratum (nodular vasculitis): diagnosis and management. *Dermatol Ther* 2010; 23: 320-7.
6. Takeuchi K, Smale S, Premchand P, *et al.* Prevalence and mechanism of nonsteroidal anti-inflammatory drug-induced clinical relapse in patients with inflammatory bowel disease. *Clin Gastroenterol Hepatol* 2006; 4: 196-202.
7. Trost LB, McDonnell JK. Important cutaneous manifestations of inflammatory bowel disease. *Postgrad Med J* 2005; 81: 580-5.
8. Wollina U. Pyoderma gangrenosum - a review. *Orphanet J Rare Dis* 2007; 2: 19.
9. Reichrath J, Bens G, Bonowitz A, Tilgen W. Treatment recommendations for pyoderma gangrenosum: an evidence-based review of the literature based on more than 350 patients. *J Am Acad Dermatol* 2005; 53: 273-83.
10. Brooklyn T, Dunnill G, Probert C. Diagnosis and treatment of pyoderma gangrenosum. *BMJ* 2006; 333: 181-4.
11. Brooklyn TN, Dunnill MG, Shetty A, *et al.* Infliximab for the treatment of pyoderma gangrenosum: a randomised, double-blind, placebo controlled trial. *Gut* 2006; 55: 505-9.
12. Regueiro M, Valentine J, Plevy S, *et al.* Infliximab for treatment of pyoderma gangrenosum associated with inflammatory bowel disease. *Am J Gastroenterol* 2003; 98: 1821-6.
13. Williams H, Walker D, Orchard TR. Extraintestinal manifestations of inflammatory bowel disease. *Curr Gastroenterol Rep* 2008; 10: 597-605.
14. Brown MA, Pile KD, Kennedy LG, *et al.* HLA class I associations of ankylosing spondylitis in the white population in the United Kingdom. *Ann Rheum Dis* 1996; 55: 268-70.
15. Orchard TR, Thiyagaraja S, Welsh KI, *et al.* Clinical phenotype is related to HLA genotype in the peripheral arthropathies of inflammatory bowel disease. *Gastroenterology* 2000; 118: 274-8.
16. Rahman P, Inman RD, Gladman DD, *et al.* Association of interleukin-23 receptor variants with ankylosing spondylitis. *Arthritis Rheum* 2008; 58: 1020-5.
17. Greenstein AJ, Janowitz HD, Sachar DB. The extra-intestinal complications of Crohn's disease and ulcerative colitis: a study of 700 patients. *Medicine* (Baltimore) 1976; 55: 401-12.

18. Orchard TR, Wordsworth BP, Jewell DP. Peripheral arthropathies in inflammatory bowel disease: their articular distribution and natural history. *Gut* 1998; 42: 387-91.
19. Chen J, Liu C. Sulfasalazine for ankylosing spondylitis. *Cochrane Database Syst Rev* 2005; CD004800.
20. Generini S, Giacomelli R, Fedi R, *et al.* Infliximab in spondyloarthropathy associated with Crohn's disease: an open study on the efficacy of inducing and maintaining remission of musculoskeletal and gut manifestations. *Ann Rheum Dis* 2004; 63: 1664-9.
21. Lofberg R, Louis EV, Reinisch W, *et al.* Adalimumab produces clinical remission and reduces extraintestinal manifestations in Crohn's disease: results from CARE. *Inflamm Bowel Dis* 2011; Feb 23. doi: 10.1002/ibd.21663. Epub ahead of print.
22. Herfarth H, Obermeier F, Andus T, *et al.* Improvement of arthritis and arthralgia after treatment with infliximab (Remicade) in a German prospective, open-label, multicenter trial in refractory Crohn's disease. *Am J Gastroenterol* 2002; 97: 2688-90.
23. Felekis T, Katsanos K, Kitsanou M, *et al.* Spectrum and frequency of ophthalmologic manifestations in patients with inflammatory bowel disease: a prospective single-center study. *Inflamm Bowel Dis* 2009; 15: 29-34.
24. Mintz R, Feller ER, Bahr RL, Shah SA. Ocular manifestations of inflammatory bowel disease. *Inflamm Bowel Dis* 2004; 10: 135-9.
25. Kim EC, Foster CS. Immunomodulatory therapy for the treatment of ocular inflammatory disease: evidence-based medicine recommendations for use. *Int Ophthalmol Clin* 2006; 46: 141-64.
26. Doctor P, Sultan A, Syed S, *et al.* Infliximab for the treatment of refractory scleritis. *Br J Ophthalmol* 2010; 94: 579-83.
27. Larson T, Nussenblatt RB, Sen HN. Emerging drugs for uveitis. *Expert Opin Emerg Drugs* 2011; 16: 309-22.
28. Murphy CC, Ayliffe WH, Booth A, *et al.* Tumor necrosis factor alpha blockade with infliximab for refractory uveitis and scleritis. *Ophthalmology* 2004; 111: 352-6.
29. Sen HN, Sangave A, Hammel K, *et al.* Infliximab for the treatment of active scleritis. *Can J Ophthalmol* 2009; 44: e9-e12.
30. Cullen SN, Chapman RW. Review article: current management of primary sclerosing cholangitis. *Aliment Pharmacol Ther* 2005; 21: 933-48.
31. Kaplan GG, Laupland KB, Butzner D, *et al.* The burden of large and small duct primary sclerosing cholangitis in adults and children: a population-based analysis. *Am J Gastroenterol* 2007; 102: 1042-9.
32. Poropat G, Giljaca V, Stimac D, Gluud C. Bile acids for primary sclerosing cholangitis. *Cochrane Database Syst Rev* 2011; CD003626.
33. Hommes DW, Erkelens W, Ponsioen C, *et al.* A double-blind, placebo-controlled, randomized study of infliximab in primary sclerosing cholangitis. *J Clin Gastroenterol* 2008; 42: 522-6.

Chapter 16

Surveillance in inflammatory bowel disease

Nishchay Chandra MRCP Consultant Gastroenterologist, Department of Gastroenterology, Royal Berkshire Hospital, Reading, UK
Siwan Thomas-Gibson MD FRCP Consultant Gastroenterologist, Wolfson Unit for Endoscopy, St Mark's Hospital, London, UK
Brian P. Saunders MD FRCP Consultant Gastroenterologist, Wolfson Unit for Endoscopy, St Mark's Hospital, London, UK

Overview

Patients with longstanding, extensive ulcerative or Crohn's colitis are six times more likely to develop colorectal cancer (CRC) when compared to the general population. Colonoscopic surveillance has been widely adopted to minimise this risk, with recent evidence indicating that this strategy has been effective in reducing the incidence of CRC-related mortality. Surveillance programmes have evolved as the understanding of the risk factors associated with CRC and the natural history of dysplasia have improved. The degree of colonic inflammation is now recognised as an independent risk factor for dysplasia and CRC development, and this has been incorporated into recently published guidelines. Pancolonic chromoendoscopy with targeted biopsies of abnormal areas has emerged as the optimal surveillance technique in patients with colitis. In experienced hands, this technique increases both the sensitivity of the endoscopic examination by improving the detection of dysplasia, and the specificity by aiding the differentiation between dysplastic and nondysplastic lesions. Management of dysplasia depends on whether it arises from flat or elevated mucosa, whether it is low-grade or high-grade, and whether it is unifocal or multifocal. Endoscopic resection and continued surveillance is a safe approach for patients with adenoma-like dysplasia-associated lesions or masses if there is no evidence of flat dyplasia elsewhere in the colon. Molecular and genetic markers for increased cancer risk are being actively sought and hold the most promise for streamlining an accurate surveillance strategy at an individual level.

Introduction

Patients with longstanding, extensive ulcerative colitis (UC) or colonic Crohn's disease are approximately six times more likely to develop colorectal cancer (CRC) than the general population [1, 2]. For patients with pancolonic UC, the lifetime risk of cancer-related mortality is 3%. Consequently, surveillance programmes using conventional colonoscopy and random biopsies have been devised to reduce this risk by allowing the early detection and treatment of precancerous changes, and to avoid the need for a prophylactic colectomy. Such programmes have limitations including significant miss-rates for small and flat dysplastic lesions, sampling errors, and inter-observer variability for determining dysplasia.

In recent times, an improved understanding of the risk factors associated with CRC and the natural history of dysplasia, in conjunction with the development of new endoscopic techniques, have sought to enhance the ability of surveillance programmes.

Risk factors

Disease extent (defined as the furthest proximal extent of either endoscopic or histological inflammation) is a major risk factor for the development of CRC in inflammatory bowel disease (IBD). Patients with either extensive colitis (up to the hepatic flexure) or pancolitis carry a lifetime risk approximately 20 times over that of an age- and sex-matched population. Most studies have found that the risk of CRC starts to increase 8-10 years following the onset of symptoms in this subgroup. Patients with left-sided colitis have an intermediate risk, which occurs 15-20 years after symptom onset, whilst patients with proctosigmoiditis are not at increased risk for CRC. A meta-analysis published in 2001 established that duration of disease is also a major risk factor for CRC. It calculated the cumulative risk of CRC in patients with UC to be 2% at 10 years, 8% at 20 years and 18% at 30 years, irrespective of disease extent [3]. This is in contrast to a more recent, single-centre, retrospective study, which revealed a considerably lower cancer incidence [4]. In this study, the reported cumulative risk after 40 years of extensive colitis was 10.8%. This lower incidence has been replicated in other studies and it has been suggested that this may be due in part to the use of chemopreventive agents, such as aminosalicylates, and the protective effect of adherence to a colonoscopic surveillance programme in which colectomy is offered to those in whom dysplasia is detected.

More recently, several studies have demonstrated that the degree of colonic inflammation at the time of the surveillance procedure is an important determinant in the risk of colorectal neoplasia. Rutter and colleagues first described this association after conducting a case-controlled study in which several potential risk factors were assessed in 68 UC patients who had gone on to develop neoplasia [5]. Univariate analysis showed a highly significant correlation between the colonoscopic and histological inflammation scores and the risk of colorectal neoplasia, whilst on multivariate analysis, only the histological inflammation score remained significant.

A family history of sporadic CRC is an independent risk factor for the development of CRC in patients with IBD. A population-based cohort study observed that IBD patients with first-degree relatives diagnosed with sporadic CRC were twice as likely to develop CRC themselves [6]. This risk increased nine-fold, if the relative was diagnosed with CRC before the age of 50 years.

It is widely acknowledged that IBD patients with concomitant primary sclerosing cholangitis (PSC) are at higher risk of developing colorectal neoplasia. Soetikno *et al* conducted a meta-analysis that included 11 studies and reported a four-fold increase in the risk of patients with PSC and UC developing CRC when compared to those with UC alone [7]. Neoplastic lesions tend to form on a background of low-grade inflammation and are predominantly located within the right side of the colon. The increased risk of neoplasia remains in those who have undergone orthotopic liver transplantation for PSC.

Patients with multiple post-inflammatory polyps and colonic strictures have a two- and four-fold risk of CRC, respectively. Whether this is as a consequence of previous severe inflammation within the colon or because these lesions harbour dysplastic tissue which is not readily accessible is unclear.

Cancer surveillance

Surveillance programmes in IBD should detect premalignant lesions at a curable stage, and ultimately reduce CRC-related mortality. Whilst prophylactic colectomy will eliminate the risk of CRC, this option is unnecessary, reduces quality of life and creates significant morbidity. However, for surveillance to be effective, patients must be willing to undergo surgery if required. In addition, such programmes should be safe, acceptable to the patients to whom it is offered, and cost-effective.

Colonoscopic surveillance is seen to have several shortcomings amongst gastroenterologists. The pick-up rate is small at approximately 11%, and furthermore, CRCs can develop even between short intervals of surveillance examinations. A recent study demonstrated that 16 out of the 30 cancers identified during the surveillance programme were interval cancers [4]. In addition, surveys demonstrate that few physicians adhere strictly to recommended guidelines, and that patients do not always accept such rigorous regimes. A Cochrane review, published in 2006, identified three case-controlled studies that sought to assess the effectiveness of cancer surveillance programs in reducing the death rate from CRC in patients with IBD [8]. Although, there was no direct evidence for a survival benefit in patients undergoing surveillance, there was evidence that cancers tended to be detected at an earlier stage in patients who were undergoing surveillance, and that these patients had a correspondingly better prognosis. Whilst no randomised controlled trials have been conducted, the evidence supports colonoscopic surveillance for dysplasia.

Surveillance strategy

The British Society of Gastroenterology (BSG) recommends that all patients with colonic IBD should undergo a screening colonoscopy 10 years from the onset of symptoms to redefine the extent of disease and to look for evidence of dysplasia [9]. As not all risk factors confer the same degree of risk, the timing of subsequent surveillance procedures is determined by stratifying an individual patient's risk. Surveillance colonoscopies should be conducted yearly, 3-yearly or 5-yearly for those stratified into high-, intermediate- and low-risk groups, respectively. The guideline proposed by the BSG is outlined in Figure 1.

Patients with proctosigmoiditis should not embark on a colitis-specific surveillance programme as their risk of developing CRC is that of the general population. Data regarding the management of patients in whom disease extent changes with time is lacking. The decision to continue with a strategy based on the maximum documented extent or increasing the interval time between procedures should be individualised to the patient. The finding of an endoscopically and histologically normal colon returns the cancer risk to that of the general population and it has been suggested that 5-yearly colonoscopies are appropriate for this subgroup.

Special situations

Despite the lack of randomised controlled trials, annual surveillance colonoscopy is recommended for patients with concomitant PSC and IBD. Surveillance should commence from the time of diagnosis of PSC as histological changes of colitis can precede the development of symptoms by several years, therefore making it difficult to establish the exact duration of IBD. Annual surveillance should also be adopted for those who have undergone liver transplantation for their PSC.

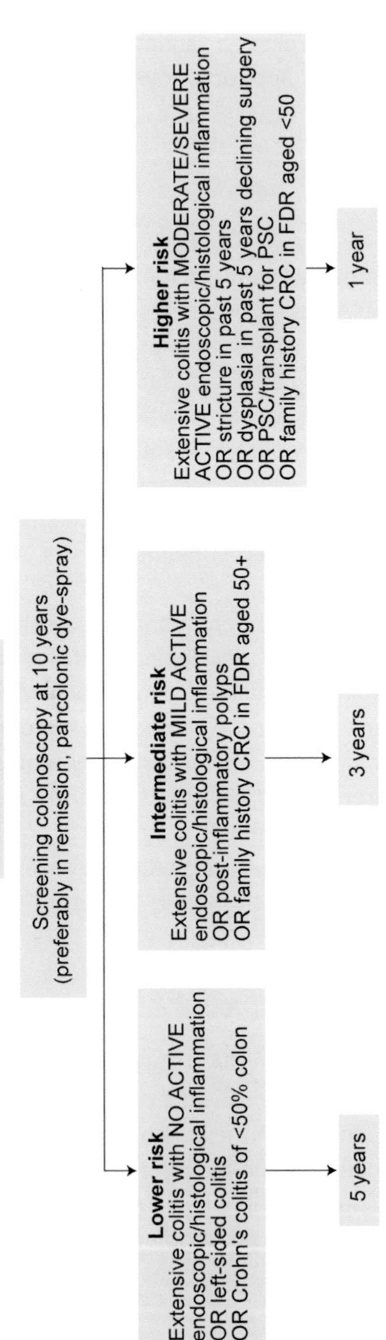
Colitis surveillance
Screening colonoscopy at 10 years
(preferably in remission, pancolonic dye-spray)
Lower risk
Extensive colitis with NO ACTIVE endoscopic/histological inflammation
OR left-sided colitis
OR Crohn's colitis of <50% colon
5 years
Intermediate risk
Extensive colitis with MILD ACTIVE endoscopic/histological inflammation
OR post-inflammatory polyps
OR family history CRC in FDR aged 50+
3 years
Higher risk
Extensive colitis with MODERATE/SEVERE ACTIVE endoscopic/histological inflammation
OR stricture in past 5 years
OR dysplasia in past 5 years declining surgery
OR PSC/transplant for PSC
OR family history CRC in FDR aged <50
1 year
Biopsy protocol
Pancolonic dye spraying with targeted biopsy of abnormal areas is recommended, otherwise 2-4 random biopsies from every 10cm of the colorectum should be taken
Other considerations
Patient preference, multiple post-inflammatory polyps, age and comorbidity, accuracy and completeness of examination
CRC = colorectal cancer
FDR = first-degree relative
PSC = primary sclerosing cholangitis

Figure 1. British Society of Gastroenterology colitis surveillance algorithm [9].

The presence of multiple post-inflammatory polyps can make the detection of mucosal abnormalities problematic. The endoscopist should be extra vigilant and if required, have a low threshold to refer to a specialist endoscopy centre with expertise in IBD surveillance. Prophylactic colectomy remains a viable management option in some cases.

In view of the high rate of underlying neoplasia, colectomy should be strongly considered in patients with colonic strictures, particularly if they are impassable. If the patient prefers a non-operative route, every effort should be made to traverse the stricture using a thinner-caliber colonoscope to evaluate the proximal colon. Multiple biopsies and brushings should be obtained, and whilst some authorities recommend repeating the procedure in a year, many advocate a much shorter time interval of 3-4 months.

Surveillance technique

Dysplastic lesions are often flat, multifocal and subtle which makes their detection by conventional colonoscopy challenging. Furthermore, histological interpretation can be difficult, particularly in the presence of inflammatory activity, which can mimic dysplastic change. Careful patient selection is therefore essential and surveillance procedures should be performed in a well-prepared colon. Medical therapy should be optimised and the examination conducted when the colitis is in remission so as to minimise the influence of inflammatory activity. However, it should be emphasised that surveillance should not be unnecessarily delayed as those with persistent inflammation are at increased risk of developing CRC.

Based on the findings of a study which found that a minimum of 33 biopsies from around the colon were required to detect dysplasia with 90% confidence [10], most authorities have recommended that four quadrant biopsy specimens should be taken every 10cm throughout the colon. More recently, however, there is an increasing awareness amongst gastroenterologists that this practice is inefficient as even the most rigorous biopsy regimes sample less than 0.05% of the colonic mucosal surface [11]. In addition to being expensive, cumbersome and time-consuming, there is an obvious burden being placed on histopathology services. The use of non-targeted biopsies originates from a time when endoscopic resolution was much poorer than with modern instruments and it has been proposed that untargeted biopsies should only be obtained if chromoendoscopy is not feasible.

Chromoendoscopy

Chromoendoscopy with targeted biopsies, in conjunction with high-resolution and magnifying endoscopes, is now considered as the gold standard modality for surveillance in IBD [12]. First described in 1976, chromoendoscopy is the technique by which tissue stains (dyes) are applied to the mucosal surface to better enhance or characterise any changes that would not ordinarily be seen by white light endoscopy. By highlighting subtle colonic lesions and therefore improving the overall sensitivity of the surveillance procedure, pancolonic dye-spraying also allows for the taking of targeted biopsies rather than multiple random biopsies. In addition to reducing the burden on histopathology services, surveillance chromoendoscopy is more accurate than white light colonoscopy in determining the degree and extent of any inflammatory activity. Recent audit data also suggest that changing in the future to a chromoendoscopy-based colitis surveillance strategy would be, at worst, cost neutral and may result in important savings both in costs and in endoscopic and pathology workloads [13].

The two stains most commonly used by endoscopists are indigo carmine and methylene blue. Indigo carmine is a contrast dye that is not absorbed by the colon and consequently, pools in depressed areas in between mucosal projections, thereby highlighting subtle irregularities. In comparison, methylene blue demonstrates mucosal abnormalities by creating a colour contrast. Whilst, methylene blue is actively absorbed by normal colonocytes, this process does not occur in either inflammatory or dysplastic cells, and consequently, these abnormal areas display a light-staining pattern against a background of uniformly blue-stained mucosa. The inability of methylene blue to distinguish between dysplastic and inflammatory areas highlights the importance of conducting surveillance colonoscopies in patients who are in clinical remission. Although there have been no head-to-head studies comparing these two stains in IBD surveillance, safety concerns regarding methylene blue have been raised following the observation that DNA damage within colonocytes occurred when the stain was combined with white light [14].

Several studies have been published demonstrating better detection rates of dysplasia with chromoendoscopy when compared to conventional white light colonoscopy for colitis surveillance. This was highlighted in a prospective study in which 100 patients with longstanding extensive UC underwent back-to-back surveillance procedures using conventional white light colonoscopes; the first of which involved biopsying visible abnormalities and taking quadrantic non-targeted biopsies every 10cm, whilst the second involved pancolonic dye-spraying with indigo carmine and targeted biopsies only [15]. No dysplasia was identified in the 2,904 non-targeted biopsies during the first procedure, whereas seven dysplastic areas were detected after the application of dye-spray.

High magnification endoscopy magnifies the mucosal surface by up to 100-fold, and when combined with chromoendoscopy, allows assessment of the crypt architecture under direct vision. Using the modified Pit Pattern Classification (Figure 2) [16], this technique allows endoscopists to distinguish between neoplastic and non-neoplastic lesions with high overall accuracy. This was demonstrated in a randomised controlled study of 165 UC patients, conducted by Kiesslich and colleagues, in which both the sensitivity and specificity for differentiation between neoplastic and non-neoplastic tissue were 93% [17]. In this study, high magnification chromoendoscopy with targeted biopsies was also three times more likely to detect intraepithelial dysplasia when compared to high magnification colonoscopy with untargeted biopsies.

Despite these favourable qualities, chromoendoscopy has not yet been adopted on a wide scale. To date, the published literature has originated from specialist centres and the technique performed by expert colonosopists. Although technically straightforward, non-expert colonoscopists will require time and sufficient training in lesion recognition to ensure that the appropriate lesion is sampled in order to maximise performance and cost-effectiveness. Dye-spraying itself can be cumbersome and time-consuming, increasing the overall procedure time

Type	Pit pattern	Definition	Usual histopathological findings
Type I	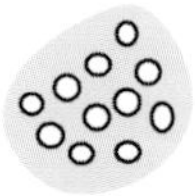	Round pits	Normal
Type II	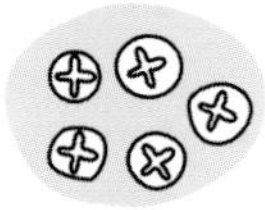	Asteroid or papillary pits	Hyperplastic
Type IIIs	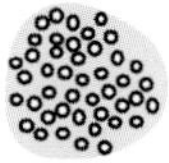	Small tubular or roundish pits	Intramucosal adeno-carcinoma (28.3%) adenoma (73%) (depressed lesion)
Type IIIL	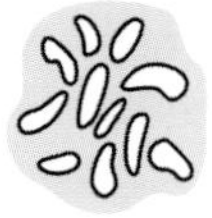	Large tubular or roundish pits	Adenoma (86.7%) (protruded lesion)
Type IV	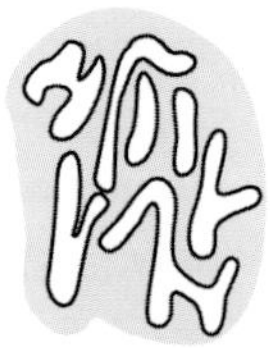	Branch-like or gyrus-like pits	Adenoma (59.7%) (almost tubulovillous adenoma) intramucosal adeno-carcinoma (37.2%)
Type V	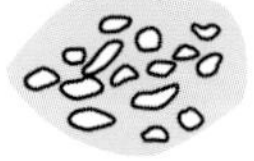	Non-structural pits	Submucosal adeno-carcinoma (62.5%)

Figure 2. Modified Pit Pattern Classification [16].

by approximately 10 minutes in expert hands. The technique of chromoendoscopy and surveillance colonoscopy is outlined in Table 1.

Table 1. Surveillance colonoscopy and chromoendocopy technique – practical guide.

Patient preparation

- Ideally perform when colitis is in remission
- Use high-quality bowel preparation regimens

Intubation

- Use IV buscopan to minimise peristalsis
- Ensure adequate visualisation of mucosa (wash adherent stool – if available use a washing pump, aspirate residual faecal fluid, use anti-foaming agents, position change)
- Biopsy any abnormalities as these may not be visible on extubation

Extubation

- Ensure adequate time taken to improve diagnostic yield
- Maintain adequate distension of lumen by position change and insufflation of CO_2 or air
- Obtain single biopsies throughout the colon to map extent and determine activity

Dye-spraying techniques

- Entire colorectum is sprayed segmentally (approximately every 10-25cm) on withdrawal
- Dye applied through a spray catheter or via washing pump
- Consider re-spraying, air aspiration/insufflation, or position change to ensure the entire mucosa is covered
- Once segment is sprayed, suction excess dye and re-insert the colonoscope to the proximal end of the segment before commencing inspection

Inspection

- Pay particular attention to mucosa proximal to haustral folds
- Look for areas of colour change or any breaks in the mucosal contour
- Assess crypt architecture (pit pattern) to determine whether neoplastic
- Photograph and biopsy any lesions and surrounding mucosa
- Resect endoscopically if appropriate and consider marking site with tattoo

Cases should be allocated a longer procedure time, even if expected to be diagnostic, and they should be performed by experienced endoscopists. It has been proposed that the incorporation of a modified foot pedal-operated washing pump may reduce procedure time by enabling the rapid application of dye to the mucosal surface whilst also freeing the biopsy channel [18].

Other imaging techniques

Over recent years, several novel imaging modalities designed to augment visualisation of dysplastic areas have been studied. Despite initial optimism, randomised cross-over trials have demonstrated that narrow band imaging (NBI) is not superior to either standard white light or high definition endoscopy for dysplasia detection in IBD [19, 20]. Data concerning other imaging modalities, including autofluorescence imaging, optical coherence tomography and fluorescence endoscopy, are limited and further trials evaluating their efficacy are required. *In vivo* histology techniques can generate images up to a 1000-fold magnification, hence permitting the colonoscopist to analyse the mucosa at a cellular level. For example, confocal endomicroscopy, in combination with chromoendoscopy, has been shown to improve the detection rate of dysplasia five-fold when compared to randomised biopsy protocols [21]. Although in the experimental phase, it is anticipated that *in vivo* techniques will allow analysis of molecular, genetic and immunohistochemical markers as an alternative to histological assessment of dysplasia as a surveillance strategy.

Management of dysplasia

Dysplasia is considered the earliest recognisable histological marker for either the future development of CRC, or the presence of concurrent malignancy elsewhere in the colon. Management of dysplasia in the context of IBD is challenging because its natural history, and therefore predictive value for CRC, is poorly understood. This is particularly the case for patients found to have low-grade dysplasia (LGD). Not all LGD progresses to high-grade dysplasia (HGD) before becoming cancerous,

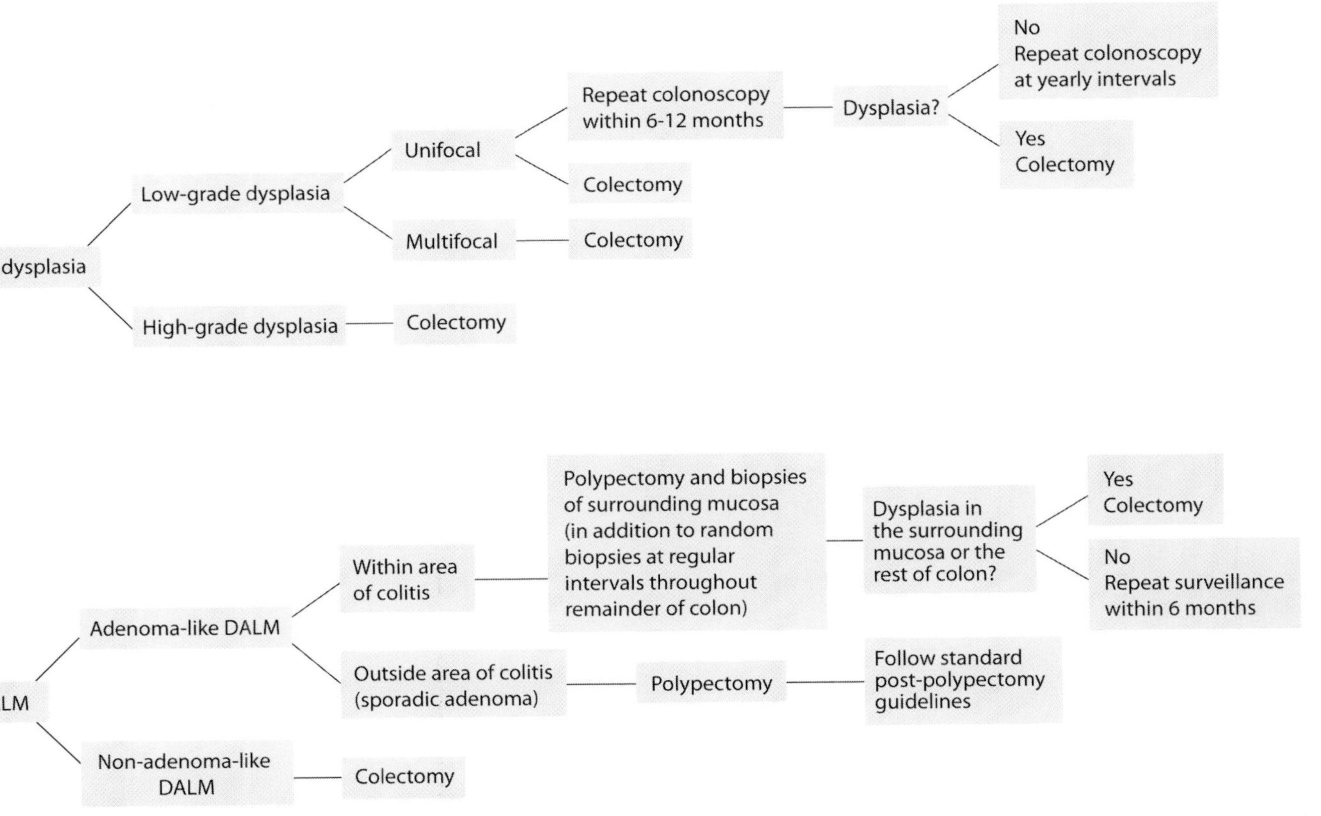

Figure 3. Algorithm for the management of dysplasia in IBD.

and in some cases, LGD can remain stable for several years or regress and disappear altogether. In addition, CRC can develop in patients without a prior history of dysplasia. The interpretation of dysplasia poses a further problem as it is susceptible to a wide degree of inter-observer variability, and consequently, confirmation from a second expert pathologist is mandatory. Once detected, the subsequent management of dysplastic lesions depends upon whether it originates in flat or elevated mucosa. An algorithm demonstrating the management of dysplasia in IBD is outlined in Figure 3.

High-grade dysplasia within flat mucosa

It is widely accepted that the detection of HGD in flat mucosa is an indication for urgent colectomy. Approximately 40% of patients will have a synchronous CRC, and for those that do not, the risk of progression to CRC is high.

Low-grade dysplasia within flat mucosa

As outlined above, the management of patients with flat LGD is controversial. Several studies have demonstrated a variable progression rate to HGD or CRC ranging between 0-55% over a 5-10-year period [22, 23]. Management options include intense colonoscopic surveillance or a prophylactic colectomy, particularly as 20% of patients will have an unrecognised CRC already present. The decision to proceed with intense surveillance or colectomy should be made with full involvement of the patient, gastroenterologist and colorectal surgeon. Yearly surveillance, even if the subsequent examination is negative for LGD, is recommended for those who elect to avoid surgery. If there is uncertainty about the diagnosis following histological review, a repeat procedure using chromoendoscopy should be performed within 3 months. Surgery should be strongly considered for those patients with multifocal LGD or those with LGD identified on more than one occasion.

Dysplasia-associated lesions or masses (DALMs)

Dysplasia-associated lesions or masses (DALMs) is the term given to elevated, endoscopically visible, dysplastic lesions arising within areas previously or currently affected by inflammation. In recent times, DALMs have been differentiated into two broad categories based on their endoscopic features: non-adenoma-like DALMs and adenoma-like DALMs. Whilst this categorisation guides further management, disease extent and the presence of dysplasia in the surrounding flat mucosa are also important factors. It is therefore essential that the endoscopist obtains biopsies and inspects the surrounding area judiciously.

Non-adenoma-like DALMs represent a heterogenous group of lesions including plaques, nodules, stricturing lesions and broad-based masses. The risk of progression to invasive carcinoma is significant (approximately 60%) and the detection of these lesions is often accompanied by a synchronous carcinoma arising beneath the dysplastic surface. For this reason, the detection of a non-adenoma-like DALM is accepted as an indication for a colectomy.

Adenoma-like DALMs are well-defined polyps that visibly resemble sporadic adenomas. These lesions are amenable to endoscopic resection and providing removal is complete and there are no other flat dysplastic lesions within the colon, the prognosis is good. Odze and colleagues reported on the outcome of 24 UC patients who had undergone polypectomy for adenoma-like DALMs [24]. The investigators concluded that, after a mean follow-up period of 82 months, there was no significant difference in the prevalence of dysplastic polyp formation when compared to a control group of non-UC patients who were treated similarly for a sporadic adenoma. From a practical point of view, the polypectomy site should be examined using chromoendoscopy to ensure complete removal, and if biopsies from the surrounding mucosa and remainder of the colon are negative for dysplasia, a repeat surveillance colonoscopy should be performed within 6 months. Regular surveillance should resume if no dysplasia is evident at this time. Conversely, if dysplasia is present in the surrounding mucosa or rest of the colon, colectomy is advised because of the high association with synchronous CRC and subsequent development of invasive cancer. Incomplete endoscopic excision of an adenoma-like DALM warrants either a further attempt at resection by an experienced endoscopist or urgent surgery.

Sporadic adenomas

An adenomatous lesion found within normal mucosa proximal to the extent of any inflammation is considered to be sporadic and should therefore undergo complete endoscopic resection if technically feasible. Standard post-polypectomy surveillance guidelines should then be followed.

Conclusions

Several recent studies have demonstrated a lower incidence of UC-related dysplasia. Whilst this may reflect better medical therapy to reduce inflammation, the widespread adoption and evolution of more effective surveillance strategies is also likely to have had a positive impact on lowering CRC incidence. Enhanced endoscopic techniques to identify dysplasia, such as chromoendoscopy, have improved detection and become the standard of care for patients undergoing IBD surveillance.

Despite these advances, uncertainty remains as to the optimal surveillance strategy and technique. Molecular and genetic markers for increased cancer risk are being actively sought and hold the most promise for streamlining an accurate surveillance strategy at an individual level. In the meantime, risk stratification based on demographic and colonoscopic features allied to careful endoscopic examination will be the mainstay of surveillance.

Key points

- **Patients with Crohn's colitis have an almost identical risk of developing colorectal cancer to those with ulcerative colitis for a similar extent and duration.**
- **The degree of endoscopic and histological inflammation at the time of surveillance colonoscopy is now recognised as an independent risk factor for the development of colorectal neoplasia.**
- **Pancolonic chromoendoscopy with targeted biopsies of abnormal areas is considered the gold-standard surveillance technique in patients with IBD.**
- **For patients with unifocal flat LGD, the decision to undergo colectomy or continued intensive surveillance should be individualised, with full involvement of the patient, gastroenterologist and colorectal surgeon.**
- **Endoscopic resection and continued surveillance is an appropriate management strategy for patients with a sporadic adenoma and those with an adenoma-like DALM without any evidence of flat dysplasia elsewhere in the colon.**

References

1. Ekbom A, Helmick C, Zack M, Adami HO. Ulcerative colitis and colorectal cancer. A population-based study. *N Engl J Med* 1990; 323(18): 1228-33.
2. Ekbom A, Helmick C, Zack M, Adami HO. Increased risk of large-bowel cancer in Crohn's disease with colonic involvement. *Lancet* 1990; 336(8711): 357-9.
3. Eaden JA, Abrams KR, Mayberry JF. The risk of colorectal cancer in ulcerative colitis: a meta-analysis. *Gut* 2001; 48: 526-35.
4. Rutter MD, Saunders BP, Wilkinson KH, *et al.* Thirty-year analysis of a colonoscopic surveillance program for neoplasia in ulcerative colitis. *Gastroenterology* 2006; 130: 1030-8.
5. Rutter M, Saunders B, Wilkinson K, *et al.* Severity of inflammation is a risk factor for colorectal neoplasia in ulcerative colitis. *Gastroenterology* 2004; 126: 451-9.
6. Askling J, Dickman PW, Karlen P, *et al.* Family history as a risk factor for colorectal cancer in inflammatory bowel disease. *Gastroenterology* 2001; 120: 1356-62.

7. Soetikno RM, Lin OS, Heidenreich PA, *et al.* Increased risk of colorectal neoplasia in patients with primary sclerosing cholangitis and ulcerative colitis: a meta-analysis. *Gastrointest Endosc* 2002; 56: 48-54.
8. Collins PD, Mpofu C, Watson AJ, Rhodes JM. Strategies for detecting colon cancer and/or dysplasia in patients with inflammatory bowel disease. *Cochrane Database Syst Rev* 2006; CD000279.
9. Cairns SR, Scholefield JH, Steele RJ, *et al.* Guidelines for colorectal cancer screening and surveillance in moderate and high risk groups (update from 2002). British Society of Gastroenterology; Association of Coloproctology for Great Britain and Ireland. *Gut* 2010; 59: 666-89.
10. Rubin CE, Haggitt RC, Burmer GC, *et al.* DNA aneuploidy in colonic biopsies predicts future development of dysplasia in ulcerative colitis. *Gastroenterology* 1992; 103: 1611-20.
11. Rosenstock E, Farmer RG, Petras R, *et al.* Surveillance for colonic carcinoma in ulcerative colitis. *Gastroenterology* 1985; 89: 1342-6.
12. Rutter MD. Surveillance programmes for neoplasia in colitis. *J Gastroenterol* 2011; 46 Suppl 1: 1-5.
13. Elsadani NN, East JE, Walters JR. New 2010 British Society of Gastroenterology colitis surveillance guidelines: costs and surveillance intervals. *Gut* 2011; 60: 282-3.
14. Davies J, Burke D, Olliver JR, *et al.* Methylene blue but not indigo carmine causes DNA damage to colonocytes *in vitro* and *in vivo* at concentrations used in clinical chromoendoscopy. *Gut* 2007; 56: 1168-9.
15. Rutter MD, Saunders BP, Schofield G, *et al.* Pancolonic indigo carmine dye spraying for the detection of dysplasia in ulcerative colitis. *Gut* 2004; 53: 256-60.
16. Kudo S. Endoscopic mucosal resection of flat and depressed types of early colorectal cancer. *Endoscopy* 1993; 25: 455-61.
17. Kiesslich R, Fritsch J, Holtmann M, *et al.* Methylene blue-aided chromoendoscopy for the detection of intraepithelial neoplasia and colon cancer in ulcerative colitis. *Gastroenterology* 2003; 124: 880-8.
18. Tsiamoulos ZP, Saunders BP. Easy dye application at surveillance colonoscopy: modified use of a washing pump. *Gut* 2011; 60: 740.
19. Dekker E, van den Broek FJ, Reitsma JB, *et al.* Narrow-band imaging compared with conventional colonoscopy for the detection of dysplasia in patients with longstanding ulcerative colitis. *Endoscopy* 2007; 39: 216-21.
20. van den Broek FJ, Fockens P, van Eeden S, *et al.* Narrow-band imaging versus high-definition endoscopy for the diagnosis of neoplasia in ulcerative colitis. *Endoscopy* 2011; 43: 108-15
21. Kiesslich R, Goetz M, Lammersdorf K, *et al.* Chromoscopy-guided endomicroscopy increases the diagnostic yield of intraepithelial neoplasia in ulcerative colitis. *Gastroenterology* 2007; 132: 874-82.
22. Connell WR, Lennard-Jones JE, Williams CB, *et al.* Factors affecting the outcome of endoscopic surveillance for cancer in ulcerative colitis. *Gastroenterology* 1994; 107: 934-44.
23. Jess T, Loftus EV Jr, Velayos FS, *et al.* Incidence and prognosis of colorectal dysplasia in inflammatory bowel disease: a population-based study from Olmsted County, Minnesota. *Inflamm Bowel Dis* 2006; 12: 669-76.
24. Odze RD, Farraye FA, Hecht JL, Hornick JL. Long-term follow up after polypectomy treatment for adenoma-like dysplastic lesions in ulcerative colitis. *Clin Gastroenterol Hepatol* 2004; 2: 534-41.

Chapter 17

Fertility, pregnancy and breastfeeding

Simon Peake MRCP Research Fellow and Specialist Registrar, St Mark's Hospital, London, UK
Ailsa L. Hart BMBCh MRCP PhD Senior Clinical Lecturer, Imperial College and Consultant Gastroenterologist, St Mark's Hospital, London, UK

Part 3

Overview

Many patients with inflammatory bowel disease are of childbearing age and ask questions about fertility, pregnancy and breastfeeding. Overall, patients with IBD have similar rates of infertility as the general population. Patients undergoing an ileal pouch-anal anastomosis have reduced fertility. Adverse pregnancy outcomes appear to be more common in patients with IBD than the general population, especially when disease is active. A careful discussion of effects of active disease on pregnancy outcome as well as side effects of medications used to treat active disease is needed. A multidisciplinary approach between the gastroenterologist, surgeon and obstetrician is advocated.

Introduction

The incidence of inflammatory bowel disease (IBD) peaks during the reproductive years. About 25% of females conceive after a diagnosis of Crohn's disease is made. Female patients frequently ask questions relating to the effect of IBD on fertility, pregnancy and effects of drug treatment and surgery on a foetus [1]. As a clinician, it is essential to have a thorough understanding of this area and be able to provide sound advice.

This chapter is divided into fertility, pregnancy and breastfeeding. However, it is important to ensure general recommendations prior to conceiving have been checked, including vaccination status, adequate vitamin levels and that the patient is up-to-date with colon cancer surveillance.

It is important to recognise that the data discussed in this chapter relating to fertility, pregnancy and breastfeeding in IBD come predominantly from case-control or cohort studies and not randomised controlled trials. Guidelines are based on consensus opinion [2-4].

Fertility

Effect of IBD on fertility

Overall, the rate of infertility in women with IBD varies between 7-12% [5,6] which is equivalent to that of the general population. Women with UC, who have not had previous surgery, have been shown to have normal fertility [7].

Patients with quiescent CD also have the same fertility as the general population [8]. Active CD reduces fertility by several mechanisms including inflammation involving the fallopian tubes and ovaries, and dyspareunia due to perianal disease.

Ideally, women should be encouraged to conceive when the disease is controlled and they are well nourished. They should take folic acid supplementation at the standard pre-conception dose (400μg/day) unless they have impaired absorption (concurrent sulfasalazine use, short bowel syndrome) when higher doses may be necessary.

What are the chances of passing disease onto children?

Patients are often understandably concerned about passing their disease onto their offspring. Family history is currently the strongest predictor of developing IBD. If one parent is affected, the risks of the offspring also developing IBD are 2-13 times higher than in the general population [9, 10]. If both parents have IBD, the lifetime risk of the offspring developing IBD was estimated at 36% [11].

Drugs and fertility

In females, the major groups of medications (sulfasalazine, 5-ASA, corticosteroids and thiopurines) have been shown to have no effect on fertility. Methotrexate should be avoided in women of childbearing age due to its teratogenic and mutagenic effects. In males, both sulfasalazine and methotrexate reversibly impair sperm production and therefore have the potential to reduce fertility. It has been reported that infliximab decreases sperm motility and morphology [12], but it is unknown whether these effects translate into altered fertility. No congenital anomalies have been reported in a series of 10 male patients being treated with infliximab [13].

Surgery and fertility

Data from gynaecological literature suggest that bowel resection for reasons other than IBD has no adverse effect on fertility [14, 15]. However, following an ileal pouch-anal anastomosis (IPAA), the data strongly suggest a reduction in fertility rates. This is likely secondary to the formation of fallopian tube and ovarian adhesions. A meta-analysis found that IPAA increased the risk of infertility three-fold compared to medical management [16].

Pregnancy

Outcome of pregnancy in patients with IBD

The majority of female patients with quiescent IBD can expect to have a normal pregnancy.

The best predictor of disease activity during pregnancy is the disease activity at conception. Seventy to 80% of UC and 70% of CD patients experienced quiescent disease during pregnancy if they were in remission at the time of conception. Active disease at conception carries an increased risk of flare-up during pregnancy and adverse pregnancy outcome including miscarriage, prematurity and low birth weight babies. One study has suggested Crohn's disease activity is reduced during pregnancy, although this may be related to a reduction in tobacco use [17]. In general, women with IBD are as likely to flare during pregnancy as when they are not pregnant, with one study reporting exacerbation rates of 34% per year when pregnant and 32% per year when not pregnant with women with UC [18].

Meta-analysis has shown an increased incidence of premature gestation in patients with CD (OR 1.97; 95% CI, 1.52-2.31; $p<0.001$) and patients with UC (OR 1.34; 95% CI, 1.09-1.64; $p<0.005$) compared with controls [19]. The incidence of low birth weight is increased in patients with CD (OR 2.84; 95% CI, 1.42-5.60; $p=0.003$), but is not affected in patients with UC.

Mode of delivery

There is an increased incidence of Caesarean section rates in patients with IBD compared with the general population [19].

Most women with IBD can have an uncomplicated vaginal delivery and this is the favoured mode of delivery in patients with quiescent or mild disease [20]. Patients with an ileostomy or colostomy can have a vaginal delivery. Exceptions to this are women with active perianal Crohn's disease or rectal involvement who may be advised to consider a

Caesarean section, as active perianal Crohn's disease may compromise sphincter integrity, which may be further exacerbated by vaginal delivery. Patients with inactive perianal disease may deliver vaginally without increased complications [20], but a clear discussion with the patient outlining the pros and cons should occur. Episiotomy should be avoided in order to reduce the risk of activating perianal CD [21].

Women with an IPAA should also consider a Caesarean section in order to preserve sphincter function and continence later in life, although a vaginal delivery is still possible [22].

There is no definitive evidence on the best mode of delivery in IBD, and the decision should be made with advice from both obstetric and gastroenterological specialists.

Drugs in pregnancy

The use of medication during the conception period and pregnancy is a source of great concern for patients and clinicians caring for them [23]. An informed pre-pregnancy (or early in pregnancy) discussion and agreement of a management plan is good practice. It is important to explain the risk to benefit ratio of medication use, and include in the discussion the risk of active untreated disease to the foetus. The use of therapies in pregnancy is summarised in Table 1.

Aminosalicylates

Sulfasalazine has been used in the treatment of IBD for over 50 years. Sulfasalazine and its metabolites cross the placenta, but are not directly teratogenic. However, sulfasalazine is an inhibitor of dihydrofolate reductase, and therefore women should be encouraged to take folic acid supplements (2mg/day) around conception.

Mesalazine compounds are poorly absorbed from the gastrointestinal tract, and there is little placental transport from mother to foetus. Meta-analysis of seven studies has shown no association between aminosalicylates and congenital malformations, stillbirths, spontaneous

Table 1. Summary of medications used in the treatment of pregnant patients with inflammatory bowel disease.

Category	Drug	FDA pregnancy category	Recommendations for pregnancy	Recommendations for breastfeeding
5-aminosalicylic acid	Sulfasalazine	B	√√ *	√√
	Mesalazine	B	√√	√√
	Olsalazine	C	√√	√
Corticosteroids	Prednisolone	C	√√	√√
	Budesonide	C	√√	√
Immunomodulators	Azathioprine	D	√	√
	6-mercaptopurine	D	√	√
	Cyclosporine	C	√	×
	Methotrexate	X	×	×
	Tacrolimus	C	√	×
	Thalidomide	X	×	×
Biological agents	Infliximab	B	√√	√
	Adalimumab	B	√√	√
Antibiotics	Metronidazole	B	√	×
	Ciprofloxacin	C	√	×
Others	Probiotics	n/a	√√	√√
	Loperamide	B	√	×

√√ = considered safe, √ = probably safe, × = contraindicated, * = supplement with 2mg folate a day

Food and Drug Administration (FDA) Categories for the use of medications in pregnancy:

A. Controlled studies in animals and women have shown no risk in the first trimester, and possible foetal harm is remote

B. Either animal studies have not demonstrated a foetal risk but there are no controlled studies in pregnant women, or animal studies have shown an adverse effect that was not confirmed in controlled studies in women in the first trimester

C. No controlled studies in humans have been performed, and animal studies have shown adverse events, or studies in humans and animals are not available; give if potential benefit outweighs the risk

D. Positive evidence of foetal risk is available, but the benefits may outweigh the risk if life-threatening or serious disease

X. Studies in animals and humans show foetal abnormalities; drug contraindicated abortions, preterm deliveries and low birth weight [24]. High-dose mesalazine in pregnancy has been associated with interstitial nephritis in the newborn infant [25] and therefore the daily mesalazine dose should not exceed 3g [26].

Topical 5-ASA preparations are considered safe in pregnancy at least until the third trimester.

Thiopurines

Animal studies involving parenteral thiopurine therapy showed various teratogenic effects (cleft lip, skeletal, urological and musculoskeletal anomalies) [27]. However, the administered doses were significantly higher than those used in humans.

The majority of data relating to azathioprine and its metabolite 6-mercaptopurine use in pregnancy comes from transplantation studies. In a recent study, the Swedish Medical Birth Register was used to identify 476 women who reported the use of azathioprine in early pregnancy, with the most common indication for azathioprine use being IBD (n=300) [28]. The congenital malformation rate in the azathioprine group was 6.2%, compared with 4.7% in all infants born (adjusted odds ratio: 1.41; 95% CI, 0.98-2.04). There was also a higher incidence of prematurity, low birth weight (<2500g) and infants who were small for gestational age. However, it is not clear whether these associations were confounded by the severity of maternal illness.

Other case series and cohort studies have not demonstrated an increase in congenital anomalies with thiopurine use in pregnancy, and the available data suggest these drugs are safe and well tolerated during pregnancy. A recent study took 215 pregnancies in 204 women with IBD in France, and found no increased risk (including congenital malformations) in women that had taken azathioprine throughout their pregnancy [29].

In general if a patient is well established on azathioprine or mercaptopurine therapy and it is felt optimal to continue this drug to maintain remission (there is a significant relapse rate in patients who stop azathioprine), it is reasonable to continue therapy during pregnancy after a full discussion with the patient [1].

A recent trial in fathers with IBD on thiopurines which compared 46 patients exposed to thiopurines at around the time of conception with 84 patients who were not exposed to thiopurines found no significant difference in congenital malformations, birth weight, premature births, pregnancy length, unsuccessful pregnancies or time to achieve pregnancy [30].

Methotrexate

Methotrexate is mutagenic and teratogenic and is absolutely contraindicated in pregnancy. It is imperative that women of childbearing age receiving methotrexate are counselled on the importance of effective contraception. It is advised that patients wait at least 3-6 months after discontinuation of the drug before attempting to conceive to allow adequate time for the metabolites of methotrexate to wash out. The same advice needs to be given to prospective fathers.

Thalidomide

Thalidomide is contraindicated in pregnancy. It is teratogenic and embryotoxic.

Cyclosporine

Cyclosporine crosses the placenta but does not appear to be teratogenic in animal models [31]. A meta-analysis examining 15 transplantation studies of cyclosporine use in pregnancy (410 patients) failed to identify cyclosporine as a major human teratogen, showing only a non-significant increase in foetal malformations (OR 3.83; 95% CI, 0.75-19.6) [32]. Anecdotal case reports exist of congenital anomalies in infants exposed to cyclosporine during gestation, but larger studies are needed to confirm these findings.

Cyclosporine use in pregnancy can be considered for severe steroid-refractory UC as an option [33, 34].

Tacrolimus

Transplant literature involving the use of tacrolimus in pregnancy has been favourable, but has shown a tendency towards premature delivery and a small increase in foetal malformations with no consistent pattern [35]. A case report describes the use of tacrolimus in a steroid-refractory UC patient as a single therapy before, during and after pregnancy with no adverse effects [36].

Anti-TNF therapies

Evidence from the TREAT registry with 117 pregnant women exposed to infliximab and from the Infliximab Safety Database with 96 pregnant women exposed to infliximab, suggests that infliximab is low risk in pregnancy and does not seem to be teratogenic [2].

The Pregnancy in Inflammatory Bowel Disease and Neonatal Outcomes (PIANO) Registry classified patients into four groups according to exposure of drugs taken between conception and delivery. The first group (unexposed) received mesalazine ± steroids ± antibiotics, but no immunomodulator or biological therapy. Group A received azathioprine/mercaptopurine ± unexposed medications, group B received biological therapy ± unexposed medications and group AB received a combination of immunomodulator and biological therapy ± unexposed medications. There was no statistical difference in adverse pregnancy outcomes between the groups [37].

A review of the Food and Drugs Administration (FDA) database literature of reported adverse events with infliximab, adalimumab and etanercept from 1999 to 2005 identified >120,000 adverse events, and a total of 61 congenital anomalies in 41 children born to mothers taking an anti-tumour necrosis factor-alpha (anti-TNF-α) therapy [38]. Fifty-nine percent of children had one or more congenital anomalies that are part of the vertebral abnormalities, anal atresia, cardiac defect, tracheoesophageal, renal and limp abnormalities (VACTERL) association. The authors concluded that a seemingly high number of congenital anomalies that are part of the VACTERL spectrum have been reported in patients using anti-TNF-α therapy during pregnancy. However, there are limitations and biases with this analysis.

Infliximab and adalimumab are IgG1 antibodies and can cross the placenta particularly in the second and third trimester. Levels of infliximab have been found in infants up to 7 months old of mothers receiving infliximab [39]. An approach is to limit exposure to anti-TNF therapies in the (second)/third trimester of pregnancy, as it is known that transplacental transfer of infliximab is low prior to this [40].

A further consideration is the risk of infection in the newborn. One recently published case report describes a healthy boy delivered at 36 weeks to a mother receiving 10mg/kg infliximab at 8-weekly intervals during her pregnancy. The infant was not breastfed. He remained healthy for 3 months, at which point he was given the BCG vaccine. The infant then failed to thrive and died at 4½ months of age. The post-mortem identified disseminated BCG as the cause of death [41]. It may therefore be advisable to avoid administration of live vaccines in infants born to mothers given biological therapy during pregnancy.

The short and long-term effects of anti-TNF-α therapy use during pregnancy are not yet fully known, but they appear safe for use in pregnancy with no increased risk of malformations being demonstrated to date. The data suggest that the benefits of anti-TNF agents in achieving remission of active disease and maintaining remission in pregnant IBD patients is likely to outweigh the theoretical risks of drug exposure to the foetus. Ultimately, the decision to use anti-TNF-α therapy in pregnancy needs to be made on a case-by-case basis.

Corticosteroids

Corticosteroids are known to cross the placenta but do not appear to have teratogenic effects. Rare side effects of corticosteroid use in pregnancy have been reported including cardiac anomalies, intrauterine growth retardation, neonatal cataracts, and adrenal and immunological suppression, especially in cases where the mother was treated with high doses for long periods in the antenatal setting.

However, a meta-analysis evaluating the IBD literature, found no significant increase in the incidence of still births, spontaneous abortions, preterm deliveries or low birth weight infants [19].

Therefore, corticosteroids can be used for moderate to severely active disease as in non-pregnant patients [42].

Surgery in pregnancy

Indications for surgery during pregnancy are the same as in non-pregnant IBD patients and include failure of medical therapy, intestinal obstruction or perforation, toxic megacolon and localised complications such as abscesses.

Historic data from 1950 to 1980 has reported high foetal and maternal mortality (49% and 22%, respectively). Recent data are more favourable. A retrospective analysis of the Mayo Clinic surgical experience between 1980 and 2004 identified five females who underwent a subtotal colectomy with Brooke's ileostomy during pregnancy for toxic megacolon [43]. All went on to have a successful pregnancy.

It is generally agreed that the effects of continued illness pose a greater risk to the foetus than surgery in these extreme circumstances. Routine non-obstetric surgical procedures can be performed in a relatively safe setting during the second trimester.

Breastfeeding

Breastfeeding is not associated with an increased risk of disease flare and may even provide a protective effect against disease flare in the post-partum period year [44]. The advantages of breastfeeding to the infant are well recognised and may include a decreased risk of developing IBD in later life [45].

Women often voice concerns about continuing medications due to possible secretion of drugs in breast milk. Table 1 summarises current advice for prescribing during breastfeeding. A careful discussion of the risks and benefits for each medication needs to occur.

Conclusions

Fertility, pregnancy and breastfeeding are a major source of concern to many female patients with IBD. The over-arching principle is that conception and pregnancy are optimised when the disease is well controlled in the mother. A clear discussion with the patient is needed to inform them of the risks and benefits of the various different medications to treat IBD, and also of the risks of active disease.

Key points

- **Fertility, pregnancy and breastfeeding are a major source of concern to many female patients with IBD.**
- **The 'golden rule' is a healthy mother is most likely to result in a healthy baby.**
- **The best predictor of disease activity during pregnancy is disease activity at conception.**
- **Ideally, plan for pregnancy when the disease is quiescent.**
- **Several of the drug therapies used in IBD have been linked with adverse foetal outcomes and therefore a full discussion with the patient, and agreement of a management plan for pregnancy, is advisable at an early stage.**
- **The advantages of breastfeeding to an infant are well recognised, but consideration of maternal drug treatment is also required.**
- **A multidisciplinary approach, involving the obstetrician, gastroenterologist and surgeon as necessary, must be adopted in all pregnant patients with IBD.**

References

1. Alstead EM, Nelson-Piercy C. Inflammatory bowel disease in pregnancy. *Gut* 2003; 52: 159-61.
2. Van Der Woude CJ, Kolacek S, Dotan I, *et al.* European evidenced-based Consensus on reproduction in inflammatory bowel disease. *J Crohns Colitis* 2010; 4: 493-510.
3. Mowat C, Cole A, Windsor A, *et al.* Guidelines for the management of inflammatory bowel disease in adults. *Gut* 2011; 60: 571-607.
4. Mahadevan U, Cucchiara S, Hyams J, *et al.* The London Position Statement of the World Congress of Gastroenterology on Biological Therapy for IBD with the European Crohn's and Colitis Organization: Pregnancy and Pediatrics. *Am J Gastro* 2011; 106: 214-23.

5. Willoughby CP, Truelove SC. Ulcerative colitis and pregnancy. *Gut* 1980; 21: 469-74.
6. Khosla R, Willoughby CP, Jewell DP. Crohn's disease and pregnancy. *Gut* 1984; 25: 52-6.
7. Hudson M, Flett G, Sinclair TS, *et al.* Fertility and pregnancy in inflammatory bowel disease. *Int J Gynecol Obstet* 1997; 58: 229-37.
8. Baird DD, Narendranathan M, Sandler RS. Increased risk or preterm birth for women with inflammatory bowel disease. *Gastroenterology* 1990; 00: 987-94.
9. Orholm M, Fonager K, Sorensen HT. Risk of ulcerative colitis and Crohn's disease among offspring of patients with chronic inflammatory bowel disease. *Am J Gastroenterol* 1999; 94: 3236-8.
10. Orholm M, Munkholm P, Langholz E, *et al.* Familial occurrence of inflammatory bowel disease. *N Engl J Med* 1991; 324: 84-8.
11. Bennett RA, Rubin PH, Present DH. Frequency of inflammatory bowel disease in offspring of couples both presenting with inflammatory bowel disease. *Gastroenterology* 1991; 100: 1638-43.
12. Mahadevan U, Terdiman JP, Aron J, *et al.* Infliximab and semen quality in men with inflammatory bowel disease. *Inflamm Bowel Dis* 2005; 11: 395-9.
13. Katz JA, Antoni C, Keenan GF, *et al.* Outcome of pregnancy in women receiving infliximab for the treatment of Crohn's disease or rheumatoid arthritis. *Am J Gastroenterol* 2004; 99: 2385-92.
14. Coronado C, Franklin RR, Lotze EC, *et al.* Surgical treatment of symptomatic colorectal endometriosis. *Fertil Steril* 1990; 53: 411-6.
15. Mohr C, Nezhat FR, Nezhat CH, *et al.* Fertility considerations in laparoscopic treatment of infiltrative bowel endometriosis. *JSLS* 2005; 9: 16-24.
16. Waljee A, Waljee J, Morris AM, *et al.* Threefold increased risk of infertility: a meta-analysis of infertility after ileal pouch-anal anastomosis in ulcerative colitis. *Gut* 2006; 55: 1575-80.
17. Agret F, Cosnes J, Hassani Z, *et al.* Impact of pregnancy on the clinical activity of Crohn's disease. *Aliment Pharmacol Ther* 2005; 21: 509.
18. Nielsen OH, Andreasson B, Bondesen S, *et al.* Pregnancy in ulcerative colitis. *Scand J Gastroenterol* 1983; 18: 735-42.
19. Cornish J, Tan E, Teare J, *et al.* A meta-analysis on the influence of inflammatory bowel disease on pregnancy. *Gut* 2007; 56: 830-7.
20. Ilnyckyj A, Blanchard JF, Rawsthorne P, *et al.* Perianal Crohn's disease and pregnancy: role of the mode of delivery. *Am J Gastroenterol* 1999; 94: 3274-8.
21. Brandt LJ, Estabrook SG, Reinus JF. Results of a survey to evaluate whether vaginal delivery and episiotomy lead to perianal involvement in women with Crohn's disease. *Am J Gastroenterol* 1995; 90: 1918-22.
22. Juhasz ES, Fozard B, Dozois RR, *et al.* Ileal pouch-anal anastomosis function following childbirth. An extended evaluation. *Dis Colon Rectum* 1995; 38: 159-65.
23. Mahadevan U. Fertility and pregnancy in the patient with inflammatory bowel disease. *Gut* 2006; 55: 1198-206.
24. Rahimi R, Nikfar S, Rezaie A, *et al.* Pregnancy outcome in women with inflammatory bowel disease following exposure to 5-aminosalicylic drugs: a meta-analysis. *Reprod Toxicol* 2008; 25: 271-5.
25. Colombel JF, Brabant G, Gubler MC, *et al.* Renal insufficiency in infant: side effect of prenatal exposure to mesalazine? *Lancet* 1994; 344: 620-1.

26. Diav-Citrin O, Park YH, Veerasuntharam G, *et al.* The safety of mesalazine in human pregnancy: a prospective controlled cohort study. *Gastroenterology* 1998; 114: 23-8.
27. Polifka JE, Friedman JM. Teratogen update: azathioprine and 6-mercaptopurine. *Teratology* 2002; 65: 240-61.
28. Cleary BJ, Kallen B. Early pregnancy azathioprine use and pregnancy outcomes. *Birth Defects Res A Clin Mol Teratol* 2009; 85: 647-54.
29. Coelho J, Beaugerie L, Colombel JF, *et al.* Pregnancy outcome in patient with inflammatory bowel disease treated with thiopurines: cohort from the CESAME study. *Gut* 2011; 60: 198-203.
30. Teruel C, López-San Román A, Bermejo F, *et al.* Outcomes of pregnancies fathered by inflammatory bowel disease patients exposed to thiopurines. *Am J Gastroenterol* 2010; 105: 2003-8.
31. Petri M. Immunosuppressive drug use in pregnancy. *Autoimmunity* 2003; 36: 51-6.
32. Bar Oz B, Hackman R, Einarson T, *et al.* Pregnancy outcome after cyclosporine therapy during pregnancy: a meta-analysis. *Transplantation* 2001; 71: 1051-5.
33. Branche J, Cortot A, Bourreille A, *et al.* Cyclosporine treatment of steroid-refractory ulcerative colitis during pregnancy. *Inflamm Bowel Dis* 2009; 15: 1044-8.
34. Anderson JB, Turner GM, Williamson RC. Fulminant ulcerative colitis in late pregnancy and the puerperium. *J R Soc Med* 1987; 80: 492-4.
35. Kainz A, Harabacz I, Cowlrick IS, *et al.* Review of the course and outcome of 100 pregnancies in 84 women treated with tacrolimus. *Transplantation* 2000; 70: 1718-21.
36. Baumgart DC, Sturm A, Wiedenmann B, *et al.* Uneventful pregnancy and neonatal outcome with tacrolimus in refractory ulcerative colitis. *Gut* 2005; 54: 1822-3.
37. Mahadevan U, Martin CF, Sandler RS, *et al.* One-year newborn outcomes among offspring in women with inflammatory bowel disease; The PIANO Registry. *Gastroenterology* 2010; 138: S-106.
38. Carter JD, Ladhani A, Ricca LR, *et al.* A safety assessment of tumor necrosis factor antagonists during pregnancy: a review of the Food and Drug Administration database. *J Rheumatol* 2009; 36: 635-41.
39. Mahadevan U, Terdiman J, Church J, *et al.* Infliximab levels in infants born to women with inflammatory bowel disease. *Gastroenterology* 2007; 132(suppl 2): A144.
40. O'Donnell S, O'Morain C. Review article: use of antitumour necrosis factor therapy in inflammatory bowel disease during pregnancy and conception. *Aliment Pharmacol Ther* 2008; 27: 885-94.
41. Cheent K, Nolan J, Shariq S, *et al.* Case report: fatal case of disseminated BCG infection in an infant born to a mother taking infliximab for Crohn's disease. *J Crohns Colitis* 2010; 4: 603-5.
42. Mogadam M, Dobbins WO, Korelitz BI, *et al.* Pregnancy and inflammatory bowel disease: effect of sulphasalazine and corticosteroids on foetal outcome. *Gastroenterology* 1981; 80: 72-6.
43. Dozois EJ, Wolff BG, Tremaine WJ, *et al.* Maternal and foetal outcome after colectomy for fulminant ulcerative colitis during pregnancy: case series and literature review. *Dis Colon Rectum* 2006; 49: 65-73.
44. Moffatt DC, Ilnyckyj A, Bernstein CN, *et al.* A population-based study of breastfeeding in inflammatory bowel disease: initiation, duration, and effect on disease in the postpartum period. *Am J Gastroenterol* 2009;104: 2517-23.
45. Bergstrand O, Hellers G. Breast-feeding during infancy in patients who develop Crohn's disease. *Scand J Gastroenterol* 1983; 18: 903-6.

Chapter 18

Screening for opportunistic infections in inflammatory bowel disease

Jean-François Rahier MD Service d'Hépatogastroentérologie, Cliniques Universitaires UCL Mont-Godinne, Yvoir, Belgium

Part 3

Overview

In an era of increasing use of immunomodulator therapy and biologics, opportunistic infections have emerged as a pivotal safety issue in patients with inflammatory bowel disease (IBD). Today's challenge to the physician is not only to manage IBD, but also to recognise, prevent and treat common and uncommon infections. The recent European Crohn's and Colitis Organisation (ECCO) guidelines on the management and prevention of opportunistic infections in patients with IBD provide clinicians with guidance on the prevention, detection and management of opportunistic infections. Proposals may appear radical, potentially changing current practice, but we believe that the recommendations will help optimise patient outcomes by reducing morbidity and mortality related to opportunistic infections. In this ongoing process, prevention is by far the first and most important step. Prevention of opportunistic infections relies on recognition of risk factors for infection, the use of primary or secondary chemoprophylaxis, careful monitoring (clinical and laboratory work-up) before and during the use of immunomodulators, vaccination and education of the patient. Special recommendations should also be given to patients before and after travel.

Introduction

The treatment of inflammatory bowel disease (IBD) has been revolutionised over the past decade by the increasing use of immunomodulators, together with the advent of biological therapy. Immunomodulators are being used more often and earlier in the course of the disease [1]. The introduction of biologic agents initiated a new therapeutic era and their use has grown continuously since their introduction in 1998 [2]. With such immunomodulation, the potential for opportunistic infection (OI) is a key safety concern for patients with IBD. Opportunistic infections are defined as serious, usually progressive infections by a micro-organism that has limited (or no) pathogenic capacity under ordinary circumstances, but which has been able to cause serious disease as a result of the predisposing effect of another disease or of its treatment [3]. Prevention of OI rests on recognition of risk factors for infection, use of primary or secondary prophylaxis, a thorough clinical and laboratory work-up before starting the immunomodulators, a vaccination program and the education of the patient. Special recommendations should also be given to patients during and before travel.

Risk factors for infection

Predisposing risk factors enable an infection to develop and progress to an extent that is not otherwise seen [3]. It is therefore mandatory to identify patients carrying such risk factors. We have defined two categories of risk: those that are external to the patient (use of immunomodulator therapy, exposure to pathogens and geographic clustering) and those that are inherent to the patient (age and malnutrition).

Viral, bacterial, parasitic and fungal infections have all been associated with the use of immunomodulator therapy in IBD. No strict correlation between a specific immunomodulator drug (such as thiopurines, methotrexate or anti-TNF drugs) and a certain type of infection has been observed. Furthermore, these drugs are commonly prescribed together, so the infectious event might be the consequence of cumulative immunosuppressive activity. Each immunomodulator carries an increased risk of infection, although to a varying degree that has not yet been quantified. The evidence for increased risk with concomitant therapy is unclear. In one large registry and in pooled safety analysis of randomised controlled trials [4, 5], no increased risk was seen, although combined therapy has been associated with an incremental increase in the relative risk of OI in one large longitudinal cohort [6] and in a case-control study [7]. Among the various immunomodulators, the use of corticosteroids alone or in combination seems to represent the higher risk [4].

Exposure to pathogens is a risk factor for OI in the immunocompromised patient. Living in an area where tuberculosis or other diseases such as histoplasmosis or coccidioidomycosis are endemic, inevitably increases the risk for contracting an OI in the normal population, and this risk is enhanced in patients who are on immunomodulator therapy [8]. Avoiding close contact with pathogens and endemic areas may be beneficial in reducing the risk of infection in IBD patients.

Although increasing age is a known risk factor for infection in the general population, this finding was not found in many series that include IBD patients [4, 9]. One single case-control study of 100 patients has identified age >50 year old as a further predisposing factor for OI [7]. It is important to remain cautious when treating this subgroup of the IBD population, especially with anti-tumour necrosis factor (TNF) therapy [10]. Malnutrition appears to be a major cause of decreased immune function worldwide and it is a major risk factor for infection [11]. Numerous factors contribute to malnutrition in IBD including anorexia, drug-nutrient interaction, malabsorption, inadequate intake, ileal resection and jejunal disease or resection [12]. Nutritional status can be measured from the body mass index (BMI) and by a formal nutritional assessment by a dietition.

Primary and secondary prophylaxis

Chemoprophylaxis is an effective and safe way of preventing infection during immunosuppressive use.

In patients with suspected latent or active tuberculosis, anti-TNFα therapy should be postponed and anti-tuberculosis treatment given, according to national guidelines. Particular attention should be drawn in patients coming from countries where tuberculosis is endemic. In this situation, thorough examination combined with appropriate tests should be done as early as possible once the diagnosis of IBD is made. The accuracy of interferon-gamma release assays (IGRA) in diagnosing latent tuberculosis in immunocompromised IBD patients is still a matter of debate [13, 14].

Primary prophylaxis for *Pneumocystis jiroveci* pneumonia should be given to patients on triple immunomodulators with one of these being a calcineurin inhibitor or anti-TNF therapy. Standard prophylaxis with co-trimoxazole is recommended (double-strength tablet daily 160-800mg three times a week) [15].

Frequent and/or severe recurrences of *Herpes simplex* virus disease can be prevented with a daily therapy with oral acyclovir or valacyclovir.

Severe strongyloidiasis may occur in patients who have lived or travelled in endemic countries (i.e. South-East Asia, Latin America, Sub-Saharan Africa, and South-East USA) during the 30 years before onset. These patients should be screened for systemic hypereosinophilia. Serological testing and stool examination should be performed. Patients with positive screening tests and/or unexplained hypereosinophilia, as well as a history of travel or residence indicative of exposure to *Strongyloides stercoralis*, should be empirically treated, preferably with ivermectin [16] before starting immunosuppressive therapy. Albendazole 400mg twice daily for 3 days is an alternative.

Severe hepatitis B flare might arise during immunomodulator treatment. In patients who are chronic hepatitis B (HBsAg+) carriers, prophylactic antiviral treatment with nucleotide or nucleoside analogues is recommended, best started 2 weeks prior to the introduction of steroids, azathioprine, or anti-TNFα therapy and continued for 6 months after their withdrawal. In line with recommendations from the American Association of the Study of Liver Disease (AASLD), patients with high baseline HBV DNA levels (>2,000 IU/ml) should continue antiviral treatment until endpoints applicable to immunocompetent patients are reached, according to specific guidelines for HBV treatment [15]. This strategy has been proven effective in reducing the rate of liver dysfunction in IBD patients who are chronic HBsAg+ carriers [17].

Regarding hepatitis C infection, no specific chemoprophylaxis is recommended. The immunomodulators are not necessarily contraindicated in cases of active chronic HCV (HCVAb+, HCV RNA+) and the decision depends on the severity of IBD and the stage of the liver disease. An acute HCV infection should be treated according to standard practice without stopping immunomodulators [15].

Clinical and laboratory work-up

General physical examination should include a search for various systemic and/or local symptoms of infection such as fever, sweating, chills, weight loss, cough, dyspnoea, haemoptysis, chest pain, cardiac murmur, dysuria and increased frequency or urgency of urination. Dental status needs to be evaluated and appropriate dental care performed. To reduce the risk of Candida septicaemia, fungal infections such as oral and vaginal candidiasis or intertrigo should be identified and appropriately treated. Gynaecological examination and cervical cancer screening should be systematically planned for women with IBD before and during treatment with immunomodulators [15, 18]. Female patients should undergo regular screening with cervical smear tests and receive the human papilloma virus (HPV) vaccine as per national guidelines.

Ideally, baseline tests, potentially performed at diagnosis should include: neutrophil and lymphocyte cell count, C-reactive protein, urine analysis in patients with prior history of urinary tract infection or urinary symptoms, *Varicella zoster* virus (VZV) serology in patients without a reliable history of varicella immunisation, hepatitis B virus and human immunodeficiency virus (HIV) serologies, eosinophil cell count, stool examination and strongyloidiasis serology (for returning travellers) [15].

Vaccination

Vaccine-preventable diseases are a major source of morbidity and mortality in immunocompromised patients. Patients with IBD are immunocompromised, mainly because of the immunomodulatory medications they take. Routine and specific immunisations are important to consider in this population. Vaccination is best implemented at an early stage of the disease. Ideally, immunisation status should be checked when the patient is first seen at the IBD clinic and a request made to the general practitioner for the vaccination record. Vaccine efficacy may not only be greater in the absence of immunomodulatory drugs, but subsequent decisions to treat with immunomodulators will then not be delayed. Vaccines are usually classified as live or non-live. This distinction is of fundamental importance because it will influence safety concerns in patients with altered immune competence. The currently used live vaccines are measles-mumps-rubella, yellow fever, and *Varicella zoster*. Live-attenuated vaccines are contraindicated in IBD patients on immunomodulator therapy. Live-virus vaccines are probably safe in patients on <20mg prednisone daily, or on higher doses provided they have been administered for a period of <14 days. It is generally recommended that administration of live-attenuated vaccines should be avoided for ≥3 months after treatment with immunomodulators has been stopped. This delay may be reduced to 1 month if corticosteroids are used alone. Immunomodulator therapy should also be withheld for ≥3 weeks from the time of a live vaccine injection [15].

A routine vaccination program should be followed in patients with IBD according to national requirements for the general population. This includes (for adults) immunisation against tetanus, diphtheria, pertussis, and poliomyelitis, with adequate boosters when necessary. Five specific vaccines should also be considered for patients with IBD. These are the varicella vaccine, hepatitis B vaccine, human papilloma virus vaccine, pneumococcal vaccine, and influenza vaccine [15]. The varicella vaccine should be considered in patients with no history of chickenpox or shingles, no prior immunisation, and negative serology for *Varicella zoster*. This represents a small minority of patients, since most of the population in industrialised countries will have been exposed to the disease in childhood. The varicella vaccine is a live vaccine and should thus be avoided in patients receiving immunomodulatory drugs. A two-dose vaccination schedule (with ≥4 weeks between doses) is recommended for adults. The hepatitis B vaccine can be administered safely in patients with IBD using a three-dose immunisation schedule. Patients treated with immunomodulatory therapy may have a suboptimal serological response. Therefore, routine testing for serological response is appropriate 1-3 months after a hepatitis B vaccination. In individuals with a poor response, an additional booster dose may be required. The human papilloma virus vaccine is a non-live vaccine that is best aimed at young female IBD patients. The influenza vaccine should be given once a year, especially in older IBD patients receiving immunomodulatory therapy. The pneumococcal polysaccharide vaccine is also recommended, with a single revaccination after 5 years.

Prior to foreign travel, IBD patients are best advised by travel medicine specialists. Travel-related vaccines include vaccines against hepatitis A, typhoid fever, yellow fever, Japanese encephalitis, meningococcal meningitis, tick-borne encephalitis and rabies. Physicians caring for immunocompromised individuals should emphasise the need for expert travel advice, including a review of vaccination status prior to travel to tropical and less economically developed countries. When possible, vaccination for travel should be started several months before the trip to allow time to assess the serological response and the need for additional boosters. The vaccine against yellow fever is live and is therefore contraindicated in patients treated with immunomodulatory therapy. Such patients should be discouraged from travelling to countries where the disease is endemic, or at the very least made aware of the risks if they cannot arrange an alternative itinerary. IBD patients not receiving immunomodulators can safely receive this vaccine.

Education

Cases of listeriosis and salmonella infections have been described in patients treated with anti-TNF therapy. Recommendations have been made to avoid certain foods such as those made from unpasteurised milk, soft cheese, cold cuts of meat, hot dogs, and refrigerated pâté, raw or undercooked eggs, poultry and meats. Advising patients to avoid eating high-risk foods when they start treatment with TNF antagonists may reduce the incidence of emerging OI [15].

(A) History
Travel or living in tropical area, history of bacterial or fungal infections, VZV, herpes simplex infections, risk of latent or active tuberculosis, immunisation history

↓

(B) Examination
Identify signs for local/systemic infections. Check dental status, cervical smear (for female)

↓

(C) Laboratory tests
Neutrophil and lymphocyte counts, CRP, urinalysis in patients with history of urinary tract infection or urinary symptoms, VZV serology in patients without a reliable history of varicella immunisation, CMV, HBV, HCV and HIV serologies, eosinophil cell count, stool examination and strongyloidiasis serology (for returning travellers)

↓

(D) Other procedures
Tuberculin skin test/IFN gamma assay (according to local guidelines), CXR

Figure 1. Screening prior to starting immunomodulators/anti-TNF therapies.

Travel

Recommendations on prevention should be discussed with an appropriate infectious disease specialist. They include travel-related vaccines, prevention of insect bites, risk of malaria, risk of tuberculosis and travellers' diarrhoea.

Conclusions

In view of the increasing use of immunosuppressive agents, patients with IBD and their physicians need a greater awareness of OI. The challenge to the medical practitioner rests not only on the management of IBD, but also on the ability to prevent, recognise and treat common and uncommon infections. In this ongoing process, prevention is by far the first and most important step.

An algorithm for screening prior to starting immunomodulators/anti-TNF therapies is shown in Figure 1.

Key points

- **IBD patients have an increased risk of opportunistic infections. This risk can be reduced with simple preventive procedures.**
- **Identification of risk factors for infection is mandatory in patients with inflammatory bowel diseases. These include those that are external to the patient (use of immunomodulator therapy, exposure to pathogens and geographic clustering) and those that are inherent to the patient (age and malnutrition).**
- **Prevention of opportunistic infections rests on the use of primary or secondary prophylaxis, a clinical and laboratory work-up, a vaccination program and education of the patient.**
- **Travel in the immunocompromised patient requires careful preparation with the help of an infectious disease specialist and the risks carefully assessed.**

References

1. Cosnes J, Nion-Larmurier I, Beaugerie L, *et al.* Impact of the increasing use of immunosuppressants in Crohn's disease on the need for intestinal surgery. *Gut* 2005; 54: 237-41.
2. Rutgeerts P, Van Assche G, Vermeire S. Review article: Infliximab therapy for inflammatory bowel disease - seven years on. *Aliment Pharmacol Ther* 2006; 23: 451-63.
3. Symmers WS. Opportunistic infections. The concept of 'opportunistic infections'. *Proc R Soc Med* 1965; 58: 341-6.

4. Lichtenstein GR, Feagan BG, Cohen RD, *et al.* Serious infections and mortality in association with therapies for Crohn's disease: TREAT Registry. *Clin Gastroenterol Hepatol* 2006; 4: 621-30.
5. Lichtenstein GR, Diamond RH, Wagner CL, *et al.* Clinical trial: benefits and risks of immunomodulators and maintenance infliximab for IBD-subgroup analyses across four randomized trials. *Aliment Pharmacol Ther* 2009; 30: 210-26.
6. Marehbian J, Arrighi HM, Hass S, *et al.* Adverse events associated with common therapy regimens for moderate-to-severe Crohn's disease. *Am J Gastroenterol* 2009; 104: 2524-33.
7. Toruner M, Loftus EV, Jr., Harmsen WS, *et al.* Risk factors for opportunistic infections in patients with inflammatory bowel disease. *Gastroenterology* 2008; 134: 929-36.
8. Kovacs JA, Masur H. Prophylaxis against opportunistic infections in patients with human immunodeficiency virus infection. *N Engl J Med* 2000; 342: 1416-29.
9. Colombel JF, Loftus EV, Jr., Tremaine WJ, *et al.* The safety profile of infliximab in patients with Crohn's disease: the Mayo clinic experience in 500 patients. *Gastroenterology* 2004; 126: 19-31.
10. Cottone M, Kohn A, Daperno M, *et al.* Advanced age is an independent risk factor for severe infections and mortality in patients given anti-tumor necrosis factor therapy for inflammatory bowel disease. *Clin Gastroenterol Hepatol* 2011; 9: 30-5.
11. Gavazzi G, Krause KH. Ageing and infection. *Lancet Infect Dis* 2002; 2: 659-66.
12. Krok KL, Lichtenstein GR. Nutrition in Crohn disease. *Curr Opin Gastroenterol* 2003; 19: 148-53.
13. Schoepfer AM, Flogerzi B, Fallegger S, *et al.* Comparison of interferon-gamma release assay versus tuberculin skin test for tuberculosis screening in inflammatory bowel disease. *Am J Gastroenterol* 2008; 103: 2799-806.
14. Papay P, Eser A, Winkler S, *et al.* Factors impacting the results of interferon-gamma release assay and tuberculin skin test in routine screening for latent tuberculosis in patients with inflammatory bowel diseases. *Inflamm Bowel Dis* 2011; 17: 84-90.
15. Rahier JF, Ben-Horin S, Chowers Y, *et al.* European evidence-based Consensus on the prevention, diagnosis and management of opportunistic infections in inflammatory bowel disease. *J Crohns Colitis* 2009; 3: 47-91.
16. Fardet L, Genereau T, Poirot JL, *et al.* Severe strongyloidiasis in corticosteroid-treated patients: case series and literature review. *J Infect* 2007; 54: 18-27.
17. Loras C, Gisbert JP, Minguez M, *et al.* Liver dysfunction related to hepatitis B and C in patients with inflammatory bowel disease treated with immunosuppressive therapy. *Gut* 2010; 59: 1340-6.
18. Viget N, Vernier-Massouille G, Salmon-Ceron D, *et al.* Opportunistic infections in patients with inflammatory bowel disease: prevention and diagnosis. *Gut* 2008; 57: 549-58.

Chapter 19

Management of adolescents with inflammatory bowel disease

John M. E. Fell MA MD MRCP FRCPCH Consultant Paediatric Gastroenterologist, Chelsea and Westminster Hospital, London, UK

Part 3

Overview

Treating younger patients with inflammatory bowel disease (IBD) is in many ways similar to treating adults. The object remains achieving a remission, which is maintained over time, with minimal side effects. In younger patients special consideration needs to be given to the impact on growth of both the disease and the therapies used. The risk of malignancy is also particularly pertinent to younger patients, and needs to be considered especially in the decision to use anti-TNF monoclonal therapy, which otherwise has been shown to have significant clinical benefits.

Introduction

Up to 25% of patients with inflammatory bowel disease (IBD) present before the age of 18 years, with some 5% presenting before five [1]. The pathophysiology of inflammatory bowel disease (IBD) in childhood does not differ fundamentally from disease presenting in adulthood. In line with these similarities, therapeutic approaches are also similar, although with certain notable variations, and some differences in emphasis due to specific features of the disease in younger patients.

Early onset IBD phenotype

Ulcerative colitis (UC) in children typically presents with extensive disease/pancolitis. Similarly, Crohn's disease (CD) in childhood tends to have a more extensive distribution than adult onset disease. Younger children (<10 years) may portray a further phenotypic variant; more frequently presenting with a colonic disease location (Table 1). Following the initial presentation where 80% exhibit an inflammatory phenotype, subsequent evolution of CD follows a similar pattern to adult onset

Table 1. Major phenotypic features of early onset inflammatory bowel disease which differ from adult onset disease.

	Ulcerative colitis	Crohn's disease
Disease location	Early onset typically extensive colitis or pancolitis	Colon: most commonly affected segment in early onset cases with upper GI often also involved
Disease extent	Early onset typically extensive colitis or pancolitis	Early onset more extensive, with more rapid further extension over time
Growth failure	(Growth failure uncommon)	Growth failure at diagnosis, reduced height velocity, and ultimately reduced final adult height

disease, with 50% progressing to more complex disease with stricture and/or fistula formation by 5 years [2, 3].

Growth failure

Growth failure is a particular concern in children with IBD (more for Crohn's than UC). This can give rise to short stature in childhood, reduced growth velocity, pubertal delay, and ultimately reduced final adult height.

The causes of growth failure in IBD are multiple and inter-related. It can be as a consequence of direct effects of inflammation on growth, as a result of therapy (particularly corticosteroids), and under-nutrition. Under-nutrition may have several related causes such as poor intake in the context of a relatively raised metabolic rate, both of which may be

Table 2. The major factors inducing growth failure in patients with inflammatory bowel disease (more significantly Crohn's disease), and the strategies adopted to mitigate them.

	Management strategy
Inflammation	Optimise therapy for underlying disease Examples: timely immunomodulation, timely anti-TNF therapy, timely surgery Timely = initiate treatment whilst growth potential still exists
Therapy	Minimise adverse effect of corticosteroids Examples: enteral nutrition rather than corticosteroids, topical (enema) therapy rather than systemic steroids, treatment escalation such as immunomodulatory therapy (azathioprine/ 6-MP) to avoid steroid dependency/recurrent relapse
Nutrition	Nutritional supplementation (micronutrient and macronutrient), may require nasogastric tube/gastrostomy/parenteral feeding Nutritional therapy (total enteral nutrition) achieves nutritional restitution and suppression of inflammation

influenced by the underlying disease/inflammatory state. Recent work has further highlighted the mechanisms by which inflammation can influence growth both via hormonal mediators, and the direct influence of pro-inflammatory cytokines on the growth plate [4]. Thus, in clinical practice since the growth pattern is so closely linked with the disease and its management, its monitoring over time has become an important means of assessing disease progress and also evaluating the response to, and appropriateness of therapies [5] (Table 2).

Treatment

A recent systematic review of trials conducted in children up to December 2006 highlighted a potential significant problem for gastroenterologists managing children with IBD, since the review could identify only a limited number of paediatric studies, of which very few were of good quality [6]. In the light of this general lack of specific paediatric data, most of the treatment strategies are derived from evidence and approaches adopted in adult practice. Fortunately in most circumstances this probably matters little since the inflammatory process of IBD in children and adults is essentially the same.

As discussed above, the impact of disease and therapy on growth is one area that needs particular consideration in paediatrics. Another is the potential for therapy to increase the risk of developing malignancy. Paediatric management also has to consider practical aspects such as the inability of younger children to swallow large tablets. In this case the availability of a 'child-friendly' medication (e.g. liquid preparation) can dictate the choice of drug.

Comprehensive treatment protocols for the management of IBD have been published in recent years: e.g. consensus guidelines devised by the European Crohn's and Colitis Organisation (ECCO) and the recommendations of the British Society of Paediatric Gastroenterology Hepatology and Nutrition (BSPGHAN) [7-9]. The treatment strategies described below are generally in line with these guidelines.

Crohn's disease treatment overview

Exclusive enteral nutrition with a liquid diet can be used as first-line therapy for CD. This is often the preferred choice given the alternative of corticosteroids. Maintenance therapy immunomodulation with azathioprine/6-mercaptopurine (6-MP) is recommended following relapse, particularly if this occurs soon after the first remission. Azathioprine/6-MP may be initiated in combination with initial therapy (e.g. enteral nutrition or corticosteroids) at diagnosis in certain circumstances. Such circumstances would include cases where early relapse is expected, for example, severe Crohn's colitis, and in cases where early disease control is crucial; for example, an older child who is still pre-pubertal or in early puberty, where growth failure and thus permanent short stature is a distinct possibility if inflammation is allowed to run a chronic course. Methotrexate can also be used as a maintenance therapy, although at present this is mainly in children who are intolerant to azathioprine/6-MP.

For persistent/resistant disease, anti-TNF monoclonal therapy (e.g. infliximab) is now established as an effective therapy both at inducing remission and as maintenance. Surgery is typically recommended for the management of complications such as strictures, but may also have a role as an alternative to anti-TNF therapy for localised inflammatory disease (e.g. terminal ileum).

Ulcerative colitis treatment overview

The initial treatment of UC depends on the severity and extent of the disease, with 80-90% of early onset cases presenting with extensive or pancolonic disease [2]. Topical treatment with 5-aminosalicylate (5-ASA) enemas is effective for proctitis, although this presentation is relatively rare in children. For more extensive disease, oral 5-ASA at higher doses can induce remission, but in children combination therapy with oral corticosteroids is often necessary. Maintenance therapy with 5-ASA is recommended as standard, whilst cases where relapse occurs early after remission, or where corticosteroid dose reduction is not possible, maintenance with azathioprine/6-MP is recommended.

For acute severe colitis, intravenous corticosteroids are recommended together with general supportive measures such as intravenous fluids and antibiotics where infection is suspected. Where this approach fails to induce a response, escalation to second-line treatment with cyclosporine or infliximab is required. Surgery, in the form of colectomy, is needed where cyclosporine or infliximab fail to induce remission. For some years this approach has been validated in adults using established colitis severity scoring indices. The recently developed Paediatric Ulcerative Colitis Activity Index (PUCAI) has now allowed a degree of objectivity to be used in decision making in affected children [10].

In more chronic cases, colectomy with a view to subsequent pouch formation may be indicated. This is typically indicated where maintenance therapy has not been able to adequately control symptoms, resulting in steroid dependency, and thus unacceptable side effects (particularly with regards to growth).

Enteral nutrition

Enteral nutritional therapy with an exclusive liquid diet is an effective therapy for active intestinal CD. In paediatric practice it is often used as first-line therapy. The major advantage of this treatment approach is that it avoids the need for corticosteroids, and thus their complications, particularly with regards growth. The mode of action of enteral nutrition is not fully understood, but it has been shown to reduce mucosal inflammation and to induce healing.

The therapy, however, has not been universally adopted (more popular in Europe than North America). The treatment requires several weeks of exclusive nutrition with a liquid diet (6-8 weeks in most paediatric protocols) followed by a period of food re-introduction. Although palatability has been improved with some of the newer polymeric formulas which use whole protein as the nitrogen source, compliance may be difficult, and administration via a nasogastric tube is sometimes necessary.

Following successful treatment, relapse has been reported to occur in up to 50-80% of cases. Strategies to reduce this include maintenance therapy which involves combined feeding of a liquid diet with normal foods, or the early initiation of azathioprine therapy.

Corticosteroids

Corticosteroids are effective in inducing remission in both UC and CD. The adverse effects of corticosteroids have been recognised for many years, particularly following chronic usage. In younger patients with inflammatory bowel disease, their effect on bone health and growth are a particular concern, as well as other adverse effects such as increasing the risk of infection. Budesonide has somewhat fewer side effects and is thus preferred for ileocaecal CD. Management strategies in general, however, aim to reduce the use of systemic corticosteroids whether by topical therapies (e.g. proctitis), alternative treatments to induce remission (e.g. enteral nutrition or high-dose 5-ASA), or more effective maintenance treatments (e.g. azathioprine/6-MP, or anti-TNF therapy).

5-aminosalicylates

5-aminosalicylates (5-ASA) are widely used in the management of UC, and to a lesser extent in CD. There are limited paediatric data as to their efficacy, but treatment strategies have been largely drawn from experience in adults. Enemas may be used for distal disease, but in the more typical extensive colitis presentation of early onset UC, high-dose oral 5-ASA often has to be administered in combination with oral corticosteroids. For UC long-term maintenance is recommended. For younger patients the nature of the drug preparation plays a significant part in the choice of 5-ASA uses, depending on their availability as a liquid preparation or granules for those who cannot swallow tablets. For older children, once-daily preparations are available which may be helpful in achieving compliance with very long-term treatment.

Immunomodulator therapy

Azathioprine and 6-MP are widely used as maintenance therapy for UC and CD in adults and children. Their use in paediatrics is supported by a randomised trial in children with CD reported by Markowitz *et al* [11]. In this study, 55 children with newly diagnosed mild to moderate CD were randomised to receive 6-MP or placebo together with conventional initial corticosteroid treatment. There was a large difference in relapse rates at 18 months between the two groups (9% versus 47%) in favour of 6-MP maintenance. Such an effective therapy does, however, have certain drawbacks, in particular its association with lymphoma after long-term use. Methotrexate can also be used in maintenance therapy although paediatric data to support its use come in the form of case series.

Biological therapy

Anti-TNF monoclonal therapy is now widely used in the treatment of CD (and to a lesser extent in UC) in both adults and children. The exact position of this approach in relation to other treatment options has been the source of significant debate, and a degree of variation between centres managing children with inflammatory bowel disease. Recent NICE guidelines (2010) (www.nice.org.uk) in the UK state that in children (6-17 years), infliximab, within its licensed indication, is recommended for the treatment of severe active CD which has not responded to conventional therapy, or for patients who are intolerant of or have contraindications to conventional therapy. It is further recommended that the need for treatment should be reviewed every 12 months.

Although much of the evidence for the efficacy of anti-TNF therapy comes from studies in adults, there has been one large randomised controlled trial in children, the REACH study, which confirms the efficacy of infliximab for the treatment of CD in children [12]. In the REACH study, 112 children aged 6-17 years were treated with infliximab (5mg/kg as standard induction therapy: 0, 2, 6 weeks). This induced remission in 58.9% and a response in 88.4% at 10 weeks. Subsequently, maintenance with a standard regime of 5mg/kg 8-weekly, resulted in clinical remission in 55.8%, and no need for dose adjustment in 63.5% at 54 weeks. The response to infliximab treatment was associated with an improvement in the quality of life, reduced corticosteroid usage, and an increase in height (reported as a standard deviation score) compared to the pre-treatment baseline. For UC, the paediatric data are more limited with, as yet, no randomised trials. Anti-TNF monoclonal therapy has, however, been used in a similar fashion to adult practice for severe and refractory cases.

Anti-TNF therapy does, however, have certain limitations. The response to treatment can be lost over time, although this can be mitigated by a change in monoclonal (e.g. to adalimumab), and the potential for allergic or infectious complications (particularly tuberculosis) are well recognised. In younger patients it is, however, the risk of malignancy that is of particular concern. Several cases of an aggressive hepatosplenic T-cell lymphoma (HSTCL), usually with a fatal outcome, have now been reported [13]. Significantly for paediatric practice, the cases were all relatively young; 12 to 31 years (and male). Most cases have occurred with combination therapy with azathioprine/6-MP, and indeed rare cases have been reported with azathioprine/6-MP monotherapy, without an anti-TNF. These findings have led to discussion as to the relative role of the two drugs in this complication, although in general there has been a more cautious approach to the use of anti-TNF monoclonal therapy in children.

Surgery

The indications for surgery in inflammatory bowel disease are generally the same as in adult practice. Thus, for UC, colectomy with a view to ileal pouch formation is undertaken where medical management has failed. In CD, surgery is also undertaken where medical management has failed, and also to treat complications such as stricture formation. The decision as to the role of surgery as opposed to further drug therapy, such as, for example, corticosteroids or anti-TNF monoclonal therapy, is in part dictated by the potential benefits of the treatments, their side effects, and risk of relapse. Growth and pubertal status in particular need to be considered when deciding on the timing of surgery. In children where growth potential remains, and thus corticosteroids may be particularly deleterious, catch up growth after surgical resections has been well described [5].

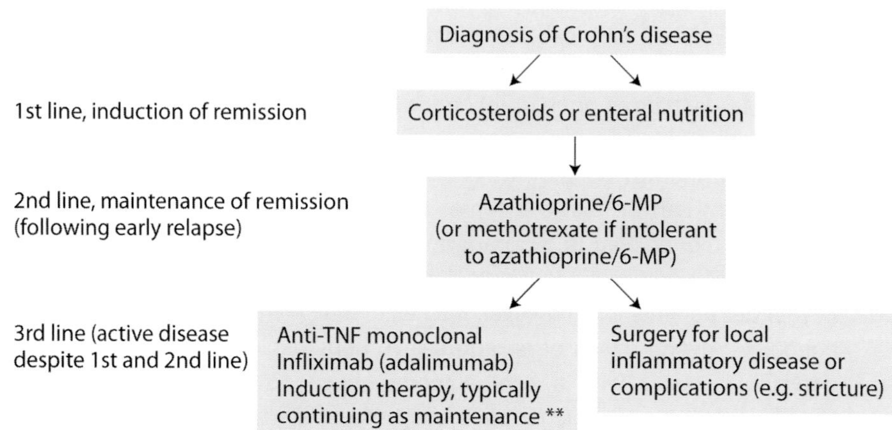

**Because of concerns in childhood regarding the risk of HSTC lymphoma following dual therapy with anti-TNF monoclonal + azathioprine/6-MP, maintenance approaches may vary:

a) Dual therapy;
b) Discontinuation of azathioprine/6MP (anti-TNF monotherapy);
c) Substitution of azathioprine/6-MP with methotrexate (anti-TNF + methotrexate combination therapy).

Figure 1. Treatment algorithm for early onset Crohn's disease, including enteral nutrition and highlighting potential concerns with anti-TNF therapy.

Conclusions

The management of ulcerative colitis and Crohn's disease in younger patients is in many ways very similar to that of adults. There are, however, added considerations such as growth, pubertal status, and malignant complications that need to be accounted for in treatment choices. These are particularly relevant when considering the fact that the early onset case may well have many years for disease, and treatment ahead of them.

A treatment algorithm for early onset Crohn's disease, including enteral nutrition and highlighting potential concerns with anti-TNF therapy, is outlined in Figure 1.

Key points

- Inflammatory bowel disease of early onset tends to be more extensive than disease in adults.
- Growth failure (and pubertal delay) may complicate inflammatory bowel disease (particularly Crohn's disease).
- Avoiding/mitigating growth failure is an important factor in deciding on treatments and their timing in younger cases, with corticosteroid avoidance a priority.
- Anti-TNF monoclonal therapy is highly effective, and thus becoming widely used, but it is associated (very rarely) with an aggressive hepatosplenic T-cell lymphoma, particularly in younger cases also receiving azathioprine/6-MP.

References

1. Sawczenko A, Sandhu BK, Logan RF, *et al.* Prospective survey of childhood inflammatory bowel disease in the British Isles. *Lancet* 2001; 357: 1093-4.
2. Van Limbergen J, Russell RK, Drummond HE, *et al.* Definition of phenotypic characteristics of childhood-onset inflammatory bowel disease. *Gastroenterology* 2008; 135: 1114-22.
3. Vernier-Masouille G, Balde M, Salleron J, *et al.* Natural history of pediatric Crohn's disease. *Gastroenterology* 2008; 135: 1106-13.
4. Walters TD, Griffiths AM. Mechanisms of growth impairment in pediatric Crohn's disease. *Nat Rev Gastroenterol Hepatol* 2009; 6: 513-23.
5. Heuschkel R, Salvestrini C, Beattie RM, *et al.* Guidelines for the management of growth failure in childhood inflammatory bowel disease. *Inflamm Bowel Dis* 2008; 14: 839-49.
6. Wilson DC, Thomas AG, Croft NM, *et al.* Systematic review of the evidence base for the medical treatment of paediatric inflammatory bowel disease. *J Pediatr Gastroenterol Nutr* 2010; 50: S14-34.

7. Van Assche G, Diagnass A, Reinisch W, *et al.* The second European evidence-based Consensus on the diagnosis and management of Crohn's disease: special situations. *J Crohn's Colitis* 2010; 4: 63-101.
8. Biancone L, Michetti P, Travis S *et al.* European evidence-based Consensus on the management of ulcerative colitis: special situations. *J Crohn's Colitis* 2008; 2: 63-92.
9. Sandhu BK, Fell JME, Beattie RM, *et al.* Guidelines for the management of inflammatory bowel disease (IBD) in children in the United Kingdom. *J Pediatr Gastroenterol Nutr* 2010; 50: S1-13.
10. Turner D, Mack D, Leleiko N, *et al.* Severe pediatric ulcerative colitis: a prospective multicentre study of outcomes and predictors of response. *Gastroenterology* 2010; 138: 2282-91.
11. Markowitz J, Grancher K, Kohn N, *et al.* A multicenter trial of 6-mercaptopurine and prednisone in children with newly diagnosed Crohn's disease. *Gastroenterology* 2000; 119: 895-902.
12. Hyams J, Crandall W, Kugathasan S, *et al.* Induction and maintenance infliximab therapy for the treatment of moderate-to-severe Crohn's disease in children. *Gastroenterology* 2007; 132: 863-73.
13. Cucchiara S, Escher JC, Hildebrand H, *et al.* Pediatric inflammatory bowel disease and the risk of lymphoma: should we revise our treatment strategies? *J Pediatr Gastroenterol Nutr* 2009; 48: 257-67.

Chapter 20

Management of anaemia in inflammatory bowel disease

Satish Keshav MBBCh DPhil FRCP Consultant Gastroenterologist and Honorary Senior Lecturer, Translational Gastroenterology Unit, John Radcliffe Hospital and University of Oxford, Oxford, UK
Stephen Tattersall MBBS FRACP Consultant Gastroenterologist, Concord Hospital, Australia

Part 3

Overview

Anaemia is the commonest systemic complication of inflammatory bowel disease (IBD). Managing anaemia requires attending to underlying inflammatory activity, correcting micronutrient deficiency, especially of iron, and ensuring adequate nutrition. The presence and severity of anaemia correlate with disease activity and is a marker of inflammation. Whilst there are multiple causes of anaemia in patients with IBD, iron deficiency is the most prevalent. The clinical consequences of iron deficiency and anaemia are now better recognised and appropriate management should be a priority. Consensus guidelines on evaluating and treating anaemia and iron deficiency in IBD were published for the first time in 2007. However, areas of uncertainly in management remain, and the evidence base for some common practice is incomplete. Issues particular to the IBD population include difficulties in defining and identifying iron deficiency, timing and choice of treatment modality, goals of treatment, the need for surveillance, and the risk of recurrent anaemia.

Introduction

Anaemia is a significant cause of morbidity in patients with IBD. It is more common than generally thought, and is associated with a reduced quality of life, increased disease activity and increased likelihood of hospitalisation [1,2]. The prevalence of anaemia in IBD depends on the cohort studied and varies according to factors such as the diagnosis (Crohn's disease [CD] or ulcerative colitis [UC]), disease activity, patient disposition (ambulatory or hospitalised), and age of the population studied [3]. Although reported rates vary widely (from 6% to 74%), pooled data from multiple studies suggest that the overall prevalence of anaemia is 17%. For patients admitted to hospital, the prevalence is as high as 68% [2,4].

Iron deficiency and anaemia of chronic disease are the most common causes of anaemia in IBD. Identifying iron deficiency is not straightforward in the presence of inflammation and the definition of iron deficiency varies between studies. Consequently, reported rates of iron deficiency in the IBD population vary between 36% and 90%. Recent reviews have calculated a weighted mean prevalence of 45% [2]. The prevalence of other causes of anaemia has not been studied in as great depth. Anaemia of chronic disease is thought to be the second most common cause of anaemia and typically coexists with iron deficiency.

Macrocytic anaemia may occur due to folate deficiency, B12 deficiency or due to the use of drugs such as sulfasalazine and thiopurines. The prevalence of macrocytic anaemia has been reported between 4.3% and 23% [5]. Folate deficiency is probably more common than B12 deficiency and is predominantly nutritional. Alcohol abuse should be considered in those with proven folate deficiency and coeliac antibodies should be measured. Medications including sulfasalazine and methotrexate can interfere with the absorption and metabolism of folate predisposing patients to folate deficiency. Patients with CD of the ileum or previous ileal resection are at risk of B12 deficiency, although the risk appears to be relatively small. Overt B12 deficiency may take years to manifest clinically because of long-lived body stores. Pernicious anaemia and other causes of B12 deficiency such as dietary deficiency in vegans can co-exist with IBD; therefore, serological testing is a reasonable precaution. Unfortunately, the Schilling test, which can distinguish between different causes of B12 deficiency, is now not available in most centres. Bone marrow toxicity with thiopurines is dose-dependent and may be partly predicted by levels of thiopurine methyltransferase enzyme. Significant bone marrow toxicity has been reported in 5% of patients on azathioprine and is probably less frequent in those on 6-mercaptopurine [5].

Anaemia is associated with a reduced quality of life in patients with IBD independent of disease activity [6]. The impact of symptoms of anaemia on quality of life may be as profound as those of abdominal pain or diarrhoea [1]. There has been a common misconception that patients with IBD adapt to lower levels of haemoglobin when the decline is gradual. It is more likely that patients come to accept their symptoms and adapt to chronic tiredness and other effects of iron deficiency. Overt symptoms of anaemia, even when chronic, are remediable and treatment substantially improves quality of life, and physical and cognitive function [2].

Iron deficiency may impair physical function even in the absence of anaemia. In otherwise healthy adolescents, iron deficiency impairs cognitive function [7], and treating iron deficiency improved fatigue [8]. In patients with heart failure, treatment of iron deficiency was equally efficacious in improving quality of life and cardiovascular performance in those with or without anaemia [9]. These data clearly raise the possibility that treating iron deficiency in IBD could benefit patients, and further research is needed to address this question.

Aetiology and pathogenesis

There may be multiple factors contributing to the development of anaemia in a particular patient with IBD including causes unrelated to IBD (Table 1). Iron deficiency is the most important cause and may have several contributing factors including increased mucosal bleeding and reduced dietary intake of iron. The main pathway by which gut inflammation results in iron deficiency is through the actions of hepcidin.

Hepcidin is a critically important peptide that is synthesised by hepatocytes and which regulates iron metabolism through its effects on intestinal epithelial cells, hepatocytes and macrophages. Hepcidin binds to

Table 1. Causes of anaemia in IBD.

	Comments
Iron deficiency	Most common cause. Multiple mechanisms including mucosal bleeding, systemic effects of chronic inflammation on iron absorption and metabolism, and reduced dietary intake. May be particularly prominent after surgery if not corrected
Anaemia of chronic disease	Common; frequently coexists with iron deficiency anaemia
B12 deficiency	Mainly in patients with longstanding ileal disease or previous ileal resection
Folate deficiency	Mainly dietary but also due to antagonistic effect of medications including sulfasalazine and methotrexate. May indicate jejunal disease, for example, with co-existent coeliac disease or jejunal Crohn's
Drug effects	Haemolysis or aplasia due to sulfasalazine. Bone marrow suppression due to thiopurines, methotrexate, and rarely, 5-aminosalicylates
Unrelated to IBD	Haemoglobinopathies, myelodysplastic syndrome and others

ferroportin, causing this iron export pump to be internalised within the cell. This inhibits the absorption of iron from the intestine, and the export of iron into the circulation from stores in macrophages and hepatocytes (Figure 1). Under physiological conditions, hepcidin production is increased when

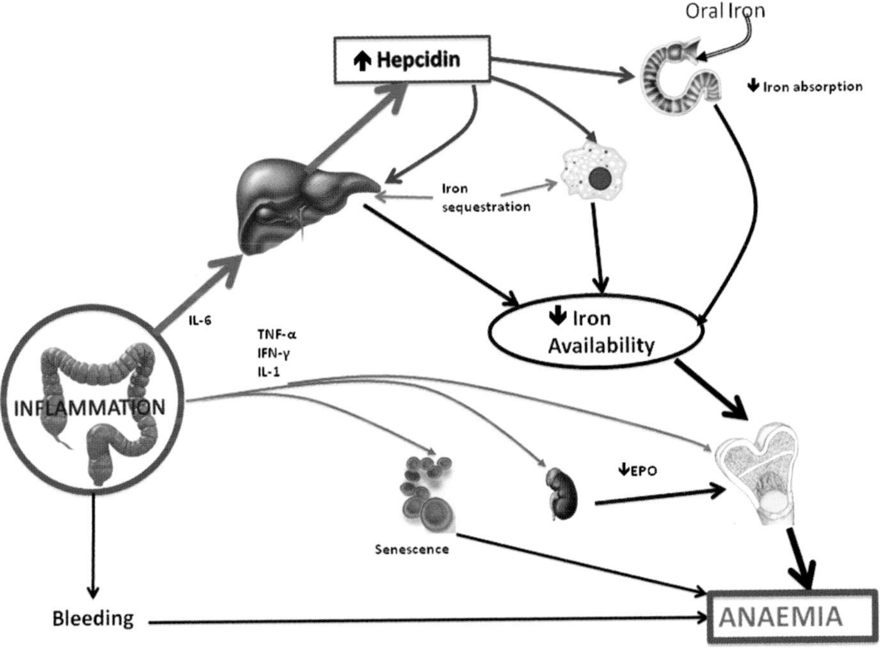

Figure 1. Iron deficiency in IBD arises through three pathways: reduced iron availability due to the action of hepcidin, cytokine-induced suppression of erythropoiesis and bleeding from the gut. Gut inflammation results in the systemic release of IL-6 that stimulates synthesis and excretion of hepcidin by hepatocytes. Hepcidin reduces iron absorption in the duodenal enterocyte by binding to ferroportin, causing its internalisation and degradation. Hepcidin may also reduce absorption of iron into enterocytes by decreasing expression of DMT-1 or ferric reductase (dcytB). Hepcidin also binds to ferroportin located on the hepatocyte (autocrine) preventing release of stored iron, and on macrophages preventing release of iron derived from the breakdown of senescent red cells. This results in a reduced availability of circulating iron for erythropoiesis. Inflammatory cytokines act on the kidney to reduce the production of erythropoietin (EPO), on erythroid progenitor cells to reduce their response to EPO, and on erythrocytes to reduce their survival.

iron stores are adequate, which reduces absorption and availability of iron for erythropoiesis [10]. Hepcidin production is also stimulated by IL-6, the pro-inflammatory cytokine, so that chronic inflammation reduces the availability of iron in the circulation, and ultimately leads to anaemia. The chronic, systemic release of pro-inflammatory cytokines in diseases including chronic inflammatory disease and chronic renal failure, causes anaemia through other mechanisms including reduced red-cell survival, reduced production of erythropoietin and inhibition of bone-marrow cell proliferation [11].

Diagnosis

There is no evidence to suggest that the diagnosis of anaemia in patients with IBD is different to the general population and therefore the same reference ranges for haemoglobin and red cell indices are applied in clinical practice. Of course, all of these parameters may be affected by variables such as chronic hypoxia, smoking, use of drugs such as thiopurines and methotrexate, and comorbid conditions such as thyroid and liver disease. Establishing the cause of anaemia and, in particular, determining iron status of a patient with IBD, requires judgement and is frequently pragmatic, approximate, and empirical. It is arguably pragmatic and reasonable to perform a check of serum vitamin B12, folate and ferritin in all anaemic patients, and in IBD, in all patients annually.

Serum ferritin is a measure of stored iron and a low serum ferritin level is characteristic of iron deficiency. Unfortunately, ferritin is an acute phase reactant and the level may be increased in the presence of inflammation. Other parameters used to gauge iron status include serum iron, serum transferrin concentration and transferrin saturation. However, these can be affected by recent diet, and may also be affected by inflammation. To deal with these difficulties several authorities have recommended adopting diagnostic criteria for iron deficiency that compensate for the effects of inflammation on measures of iron status. A serum ferritin $<30\mu g/L$ or transferrin saturation $<16\%$ are regarded as diagnostic of iron deficiency in those without clinical or biochemical evidence of inflammation. In the presence of inflammation a higher threshold of serum ferritin is appropriate.

The published guidelines recommend increasing the threshold to 100µg/L in the presence of inflammation [12]. However, many patients are iron-deficient even with a serum ferritin >100µg/L. The clinician should think of probability of iron deficiency falling with increasing ferritin, and the level of confidence varies with the exact value of the ferritin, and the intensity of inflammation. Unfortunately, a nomogram to reliably calculate exact levels of confidence has yet to be devised (Figure 2). Pragmatically, we would only consider iron deficiency excluded in active IBD with a serum ferritin level >1000µg/L.

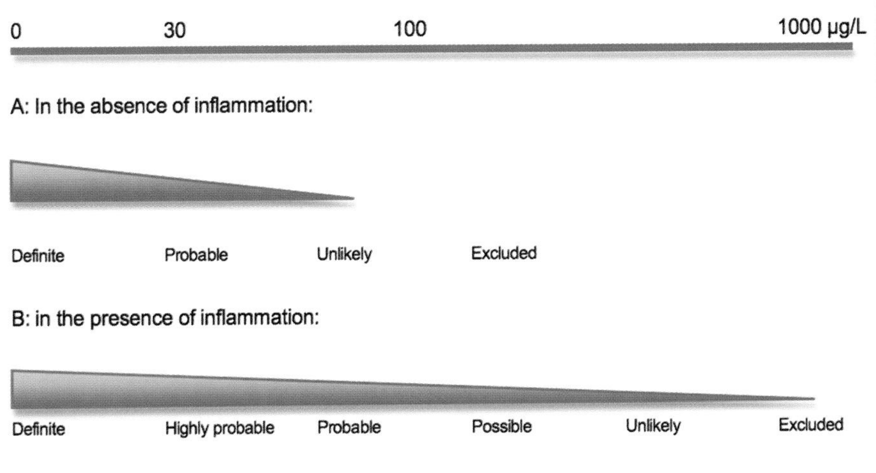

Figure 2. Probability of iron deficiency according to serum ferritin.

Other approaches to distinguishing iron deficiency anaemia from anaemia of chronic disease include measuring the soluble transferrin receptor (sTfR) level in serum, sTfR to ferritin ratio, bone marrow biopsy, liver biopsy and diagnostic trial of iron (Table 2). The difficulty with assessing the value of new measures of iron status is that there is no gold standard against which to measure them. Bone marrow biopsy and liver

Table 2. Common diagnostic tests.

Test	Interpretation	Advantages	Limitations
Red cell indices	MCV <70, MCH <30 compatible with iron deficiency	Simple and widely available	Affected by medications (AZA), other micronutrients (B12, folate) and other factors (alcohol intake, thyroid status, haemoglobinopathies)
Ferritin	Ferritin <30µg/L very specific for iron deficiency. Rises during inflammation. Probability of iron deficiency falls with increasing ferritin	Simple, widely available Most accurate test Partially predictable response to inflammation	Interpretation affected by presence of inflammation, liver disease, malignancy
Serum iron	Reduced in presence of iron deficiency (and inflammation)	Widely available	Poor reflection of iron stores. Varies substantially with recent diet. Difficult to interpret in presence of inflammation
Serum transferrin (total iron binding capacity)	Increased in presence of iron deficiency	Widely available	An indirect measure of iron stores. Less accurate than ferritin
Transferrin saturation	Reduced in iron deficiency. In absence of inflammation <16% diagnostic of iron deficiency	Widely available	Useful in the absence of inflammation but difficult to interpret when active inflammation present

Table 2. Common diagnostic tests *continued.*

Test	Interpretation	Advantages	Limitations
Soluble transferrin receptor	Increased in iron deficiency	Less susceptible to inflammation than other 'iron studies'. May be useful adjunct to ferritin with sTfR/ferritin ratio	Not widely available, not proven to have better accuracy than ferritin in IBD
Bone marrow or liver biopsy	Sometimes considered gold standard test Absence of stainable iron highly specific	Accurate	Invasive
Diagnostic trial of iron	Reticulocytosis over 5-7 days followed by improvement in Hb and red cell indices over 2-4 weeks	Therapeutic as well as diagnostic	Absorption of oral iron unreliable in IBD and affected by inflammation. IV iron relatively expensive. Risk of treating patients without iron deficiency is probably insignificant

MCV = mean corpuscular volume; MCH = mean corpuscular haemoglobin

biopsy with biochemical estimates of iron stores are regarded as close markers for total body iron stores; however, they are unsuitable for clinical practice. sTfR is released from erythropoietic precursor cells in the bone marrow, and rising levels indicate an increased requirement for iron in these cells [13]. Therefore, serum sTfR levels are an indirect measure of iron deficiency, and seem to be unaffected by inflammation. The sTfR to ferritin ratio appears to perform even more robustly as a test of iron deficiency, although neither test has been applied directly to the IBD population [14]. Currently the sTfR assay is expensive and not generally available.

Where diagnostic tests remain equivocal and clinical suspicion remains high, a diagnostic trial of iron therapy may be appropriate and unavoidable. Reticulocytosis after 3-5 days and an increase in haemoglobin at 2-4 weeks confirm the diagnosis.

The diagnosis of folate and vitamin B12 deficiency may also be complicated. In the presence of macrocytosis, the first step is measurement of serum levels of both folate and B12. Serum folate levels are affected acutely by diet, and red-cell folate levels are a more accurate reflection of stores. However, this test is more expensive and has other limitations. Serum cobalamin measurement is also subject to variation, and can be affected by diet and inflammation. Despite this, B12 deficiency is unlikely in the presence of serum levels >220pmol/L and moderately likely with levels <135pmol/L [15]. Repeated measurement of B12 may be helpful to guide therapy. However, if there is high clinical suspicion of B12 deficiency, supported by observed macrocytosis, hypersegmentation of neutrophils or symptoms of deficiency such as paraesthesia and fatigue, intramuscular replacement therapy and repeat measurement is reasonable. Elevated levels of serum homocysteine and methylmalonic acid may help to support the diagnosis in these cases.

Clinicians should be vigilant about detecting anaemia in patients with IBD and have a low threshold for checking iron status and for other nutrient deficiencies. In patients with quiescent disease, iron status should be checked annually, more frequently in those with active disease. If the cause of anaemia is not evident from initial testing, then the other causes listed in Table 1 should be considered and, where appropriate, tested for. For those in whom the cause remains elusive then referral to haematology should be considered.

Treatment

The presence and severity of anaemia in patients with IBD correlates with disease activity and so a key aspect of treating anaemia is to control the underlying disease. In most cases anaemia will not be controlled in the long term if IBD remains active.

Folate deficiency

Folate deficiency can be treated with oral supplementation (usually 1-5mg folic acid daily) as in patients without IBD. Co-existent B12 deficiency should always be checked for before treating folate deficiency due to the risk of irreversibly worsening neurological symptoms. After successful treatment patients should be monitored for recurrence, particularly if the underlying disease remains active. Nutritional assessment and advice may be helpful if dietary intake is inadequate and excessive alcohol use (when present) should be addressed. Commercially available multivitamins contain adequate doses of folate (>200μg/day) to avoid recurrence in most cases.

Vitamin B12 deficiency

B12 deficiency should be initially treated with intramuscular injections of hydroxocobalamin. A typical schedule would be 1mg per day for 1 week, followed by further injections at weekly intervals, to achieve a total dose of 6-10mg over 6 weeks. Haematological and neurological response should be assessed and further doses may be warranted. Most patients will require life-long maintenance treatment with 1mg hydroxocobalamin every 12 weeks if deficiency is caused by ileal resection or pernicious anaemia. Deficiency of folate and B12 may cause hyperhomocysteinaemia which is a risk factor for thrombosis, further justifying assiduous correction of deficiency.

Iron deficiency

Mild iron deficiency anaemia, although common, should not be unquestioningly tolerated in patients with IBD. The goal of treatment should be to achieve a normal haemoglobin with completely replenished iron stores. Recurrent iron deficiency is common, and in a recent study, over half of all patients developed recurrent anaemia after 10 months following adequate treatment of iron deficiency [16]. When iron deficiency is corrected, iron stores are usually assessed by measuring the serum ferritin level. The risk of recurrence is inversely proportional to the maximum ferritin level achieved with treatment. The target ferritin level should be at least 100µg/L, and a higher level, such as >400µg/L, may reduce the rate of recurrence.

Oral and parenteral iron replacement

Iron replacement may be given with oral or intravenous (IV) preparations. Intramuscular iron is largely obsolete because absorption is unreliable, the doses administered relatively small and side effects including pain and skin discolouration are common. Blood transfusions may be required in some circumstances when there is haemodynamic compromise or a need to rapidly increase oxygen delivery to tissues; however, this has many disadvantages including cost and the risk of adverse effects. Blood transfusions should not be used simply to treat iron deficiency. Oral iron formulations are cheap, convenient, widely available, and effective for the majority of patients with IBD [17]. In clinical trials of oral iron in IBD, 20-30% of patients stop treatment due to side effects [18]. This rate is not substantially different to that observed in the general population, although it may be an underestimate as patients with known intolerance are usually excluded from participation in trials. In animal models, oral iron supplementation is associated with increased intestinal oxidative stress, inflammation and disease activity [19]. In humans, however, although there is some evidence of increased oxidative stress, oral iron seems to be safe and effective with little evidence of increased activity of underlying IBD [18, 20, 21].

Several formulations of oral iron are available, containing the ferrous (Fe++) ionic form with sulphate, fumarate, or gluconate. Ferric iron is poorly absorbed, and is not commercially available for treatment. The amount of elemental iron per gram differs in each formulation, and when this is corrected for, there are no substantial differences in side effects, efficacy or tolerability between the various salt forms (Table 3). Doses of 200mg of elemental iron per day (equivalent to three 200mg tablets of ferrous sulphate) are commonly used to treat iron deficiency. The absorption of iron via duodenal enterocytes is tightly regulated and saturable, therefore, doses that exceed this absorptive capacity do not offer any benefit, and are associated with a higher risk of intolerance. In

Table 3. Iron content of oral iron preparations.

Oral iron preparation	Typical tablet size	Elemental iron content	Recommended dose
Ferrous sulphate	200mg	60mg	2 x 200mg tablets daily
Ferrous gluconate	300mg	35mg	3 x 300mg tablets daily
Ferrous fumarate	200mg	65mg	2 x 200mg tablets daily

the absence of IBD, for example, in elderly patients and pregnant women with iron deficiency, doses as low as 30mg of elemental iron per day are as effective as larger doses, and are associated with fewer side effects. Patients with IBD who are iron deficient should be treated with no more than 100mg of elemental iron per day orally. It may take 6 months or more of continuous oral treatment to replenish iron stores in patients with IBD, and this rate cannot be increased by increasing the daily dose. Iron absorption is reduced during periods of active disease in patients with IBD [22] and in some cases the rate of iron loss exceeds the capacity of the duodenum to absorb iron so that oral replacement is completely ineffective. The haematological and biochemical response to treatment should be assessed with repeat measurement of haemoglobin and ferritin after 4-6 weeks and if the response is suboptimal, treatment should be switched to an intravenous route.

In the context of IBD, intravenous iron is probably more effective than oral iron at correcting anaemia and replenishing iron stores when tolerability and compliance are taken into consideration. For this reason, IV iron is recommended in active IBD where feasible. However, oral iron is non-invasive and cheaper, and does not require the support of infrastructure such as an infusion centre, nursing and pharmacy support that may only be available in secondary care and specialist centres. Therefore, the use of oral iron when there are no specific contraindications is also a reasonable option. Serious reactions to intravenous iron therapy were common when high-molecular-weight iron-dextran complexes were the only available option. These formulations, which carried the risk of life-threatening anaphylactic reactions, renal damage, and dose-dependent iron toxicity should now be regarded as obsolete. Several modern intravenous iron formulations with differences in the dosing and side-effect profiles are now available. Serious adverse events are extremely uncommon with newer formulations such as low-molecular-weight iron dextran (LMWID), iron gluconate, iron sucrose, ferric carboxymaltose and iron isomaltoside.

The formulations differ according to the size of the dose that can be administered, the need for a test dose and the time needed to complete infusion. When undertaking treatment with intravenous iron supplements it is worthwhile calculating a total iron deficit to guide dosing. The Ganzoni formula (below) is widely used for this purpose. For a man of average weight with mild-moderate anaemia, a typical iron deficit is 1000-1500mg. Higher doses of iron can be given with LMWID (total-dose infusion), iron isomaltoside (20mg/kg) and ferric carboxymaltose (15mg/kg) such that in the majority of patients total-dose iron infusions can be given in a single sitting. For the other formulations a schedule of repeated infusions over several weeks is usually required.

The Ganzoni equation:

Total iron deficit = Body weight (kg) x (target Hb - actual Hb) (g/dL) x 2.4 + iron stores* (mg)

* Iron stores are commonly estimated as 500mg

There is considerable experience with iron sucrose including trials demonstrating superiority to oral iron in patients with IBD [20, 21, 23]. Iron sucrose has the best safety record of any IV iron preparation, although it has the disadvantage of being limited to infusions of 200-500mg at a time, and 600mg/week, so that typically 5-10 infusions are required over a period of several weeks to replace the total iron deficit. Ferric carboxymaltose can be administered in doses up to 1g (15mg/kg) per infusion, and has demonstrated efficacy in patients with IBD [24]. A recent head-to-head comparison of ferric carboxymaltose with iron sucrose in patients with IBD found a higher rate of response at 12 weeks with ferric-

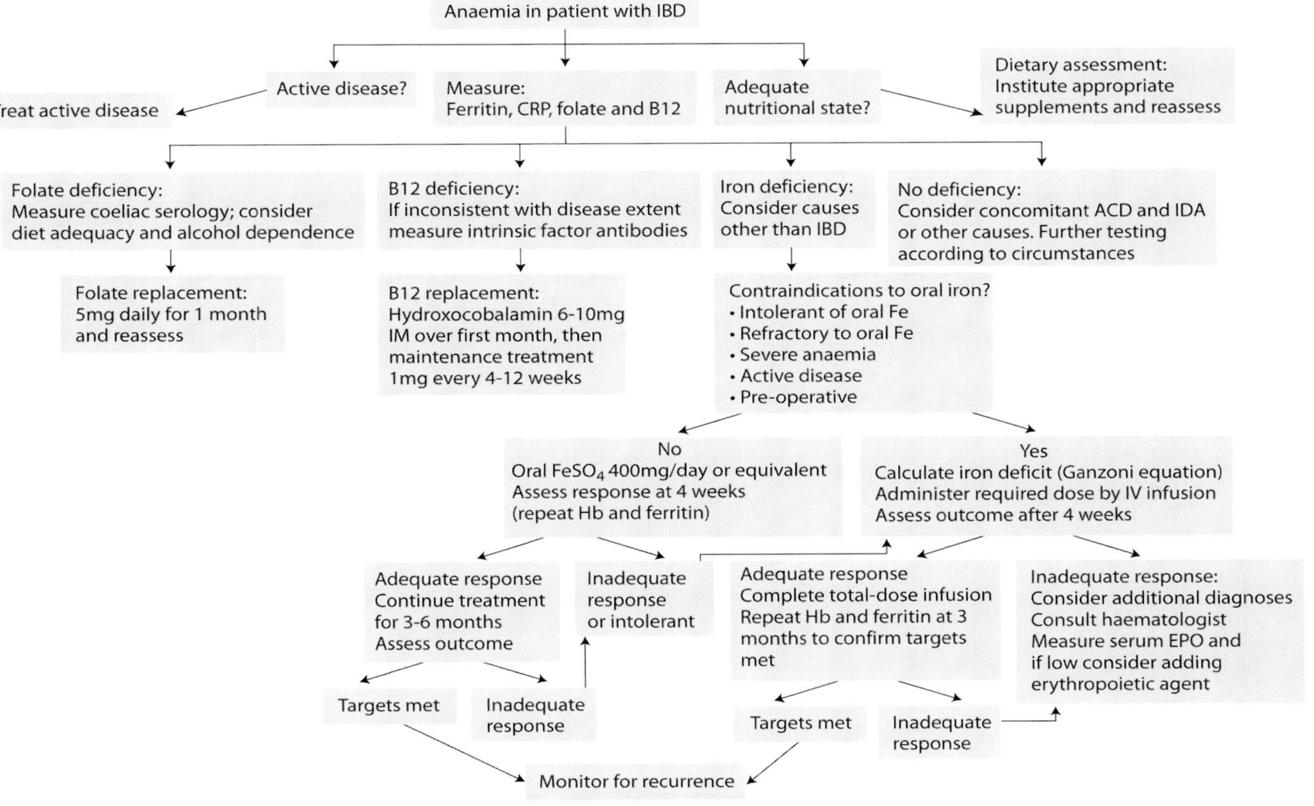

Figure 3. Treatment algorithm for the management of anaemia in inflammatory bowel disease.

Part 3

carboxymaltose [25]. This was achieved with fewer infusions, although there was a statistically non-significant excess of adverse events in those treated with ferric carboxymaltose. Ferric carboxymaltose is widely used in Europe and the UK; however, it has not been approved for use in the USA. LMWID is safe and effective in delivering total-dose iron replacement in a single infusion in patients with IBD. A test dose is required before infusion of LMWID. A significant minority of patients (8%) will react to a test dose and they should not proceed to receive a total-dose infusion [26].

Intravenous iron should be preferred in patients with severe iron deficiency anaemia (Hb <10g/dL), patients with active inflammation, for anaemia refractory to oral iron, in patients intolerant of oral iron, and in those in whom rapid correction of iron stores is advantageous (such as pre-operative patients). More than 70% of patients treated with intravenous iron have an adequate response. For those who do not respond, a search for occult inflammation or bleeding should be undertaken. Other causes of anaemia including haemolysis and myelodysplastic syndrome should be considered and in some circumstances a referral to a haematologist may be helpful. The addition of erythropoietic agents in patients with anaemia refractory to intravenous iron supplementation may increase the response. This may be particularly true in the presence of low circulating levels of erythropoietin [27]. Treatment with erythropoietic agents should be reserved for those who would otherwise require transfusion and, in our experience, is rarely required.

A treatment algorithm for the management of anaemia in inflammatory bowel disease is shown in Figure 3.

Neglected issues and unanswered questions

The interaction between chronic intestinal inflammation and iron absorption and metabolism is complex. Even low-grade intestinal inflammation such as that seen in the ileoanal pouch may be sufficient to cause iron deficiency [28]. Although anaemia is a common problem in other chronic inflammatory conditions such as rheumatoid arthritis, it does not appear to be of the same magnitude as for patients with IBD. Whilst some of this may be attributed to mucosal bleeding there may be features of inflammation in the gut that have a unique impact on iron metabolism.

Iron deficiency anaemia is a common problem after surgery for inflammatory bowel disease resulting in morbidity and delayed recovery. In patients scheduled for surgery who are anaemic or who have borderline iron reservoirs, pre-operative iron infusions are an attractive option allowing rapid replenishment of iron stores. Oral iron may be difficult to administer in this setting and is unlikely to be as effective. Studies are needed to assess the efficacy of intravenous iron in this setting.

Patients with iron deficiency and normal haemoglobin are frequently encountered in IBD clinics. These patients are often not treated because oral iron is poorly tolerated and the use of intravenous preparations would not have been considered justified. There is accumulating evidence that iron deficiency by itself is associated with morbidity; therefore, whether or not these patients should be treated, and how this would affect quality of life and disease activity are important unanswered questions. Pre-clinical studies of the pro-inflammatory effects of iron raise the prospect of worsening disease activity when iron is administered. However, high doses of intravenous iron may actually decrease inflammation by down-regulating pro-inflammatory signalling by macrophages. In several trials in IBD there has been a trend to reduced disease activity scores with treatment (both oral and IV).

Conclusions

Anaemia is a major cause of morbidity in patients with IBD. Anaemia is associated with hospitalisation, reduced quality of life and reduced physiological functioning. The major risk factor for anaemia is active inflammation, which is associated with mucosal bleeding and an inflammatory cascade that results in reduced systemic availability of iron and reduced erythropoiesis. The commonest causes of anaemia in IBD are iron deficiency and anaemia of chronic disease. Evaluation of the anaemic patient should include an assessment of iron stores taking into account the presence of systemic inflammation. The treatment of anaemia should include controlling inflammation, correcting micronutrient deficiencies, and anticipating recurrence. Although oral iron is effective, modern intravenous preparations of iron offer many advantages that may be particularly relevant in IBD.

Key points

- The optimum treatment of anaemia in IBD includes controlling inflammation, replenishing deficient micronutrients, and ensuring adequate nutrition.
- Anaemia is common in patients with IBD – and is the most common extraintestinal manifestation. Iron deficiency and anaemia of chronic disease are the main cause.
- Treatment should aim to normalise haemoglobin and replenish stores of iron, B12, and folate to prevent rapid recurrence.
- After treatment, patients risk recurrent anaemia and iron deficiency. They should be closely monitored and re-treated as necessary.
- Oral iron replacement is safe and effective. However, it is poorly tolerated, and patients may not adhere to prescriptions. The dose of oral iron used should be equivalent to 100mg of elemental iron per day, which is the limit of what can be absorbed, and is better tolerated than higher doses.
- Newer intravenous iron preparations are safe, efficacious and well tolerated. Intravenous replacement is preferred for patients with severe anaemia and those with active, symptomatic inflammation, as well as in patients who are refractory to oral therapy.
- Vitamin B12 usually needs to be replenished by intramuscular injection unless the cause is dietary.
- Folate is usually replaced by oral supplementation.

References

1. Gasche C, Lomer MC, Cavill I, Weiss G. Iron, anaemia, and inflammatory bowel diseases. *Gut* 2004; 53: 1190-7.
2. Gomollon F, Gisbert JP. Anemia and inflammatory bowel diseases. *World J Gastroenterol* 2009; 15(37): 4659-65.

3. Wilson A, Reyes E, Ofman J. Prevalence and outcomes of anemia in inflammatory bowel disease: a systematic review of the literature. *Am J Med* 2004; 116 Suppl 7A: 44S-9.
4. Voegtlin M, Vavricka SR, Schoepfer AM, *et al.* Prevalence of anaemia in inflammatory bowel disease in Switzerland: a cross-sectional study in patients from private practices and university hospitals. *J Crohns Colitis* 2010; 4: 642-8.
5. Kulnigg S, Gasche C. Systematic review: managing anaemia in Crohn's disease. *Aliment Pharmacol Ther* 2006; 24(11-12): 1507-23.
6. Wells CW, Lewis S, Barton JR, Corbett S. Effects of changes in hemoglobin level on quality of life and cognitive function in inflammatory bowel disease patients. *Inflamm Bowel Dis* 2006; 12: 123-30.
7. Bruner AB, Joffe A, Duggan AK, *et al.* Randomised study of cognitive effects of iron supplementation in non-anaemic iron-deficient adolescent girls. *Lancet* 1996; 348(9033): 992-6.
8. Verdon F, Burnand B, Stubi CL, *et al.* Iron supplementation for unexplained fatigue in non-anaemic women: double-blind randomised placebo-controlled trial. *BMJ* 2003; 326(7399): 1124.
9. Anker SD, Comin Colet J, Filippatos G, *et al.* Ferric carboxymaltose in patients with heart failure and iron deficiency. *N Engl J Med* 2009; 361(25): 2436-48.
10. Fleming RE, Bacon BR. Orchestration of iron homeostasis. *N Engl J Med* 2005; 352(17): 1741-4.
11. Weiss G, Goodnough LT. Anemia of chronic disease. *N Engl J Med* 2005; 352(10): 1011-23.
12. Gasche C, Berstad A, Befrits R, *et al.* Guidelines on the diagnosis and management of iron deficiency and anemia in inflammatory bowel diseases. *Inflamm Bowel Dis* 2007; 13(12): 1545-53.
13. Koulaouzidis A, Said E, Cottier R, Saeed AA. Soluble transferrin receptors and iron deficiency, a step beyond ferritin. A systematic review. *J Gastrointestin Liver Dis* 2009; 18: 345-52.
14. Pettersson T, Kivivuori SM, Siimes MA. Is serum transferrin receptor useful for detecting iron-deficiency in anaemic patients with chronic inflammatory diseases? *Br J Rheumatol* 1994; 33: 740-4.
15. Dali-Youcef N, Andres E. An update on cobalamin deficiency in adults. *QJM* 2009; 102: 17-28.
16. Kulnigg S, Teischinger L, Dejaco C, *et al.* Rapid recurrence of IBD-associated anemia and iron deficiency after intravenous iron sucrose and erythropoietin treatment. *Am J Gastroenterol* 2009; 104: 1460-7.
17. Munoz M, Gomez-Ramirez S, Garcia-Erce JA. Intravenous iron in inflammatory bowel disease. *World J Gastroenterol* 2009; 15(37): 4666-74.
18. de Silva AD, Tsironi E, Feakins RM, Rampton DS. Efficacy and tolerability of oral iron therapy in inflammatory bowel disease: a prospective, comparative trial. *Aliment Pharmacol Ther* 2005; 22(11-12): 1097-105.
19. Aghdassi E, Carrier J, Cullen J, *et al.* Effect of iron supplementation on oxidative stress and intestinal inflammation in rats with acute colitis. *Dig Dis Sci* 2001; 46: 1088-94.

20. Schroder O, Mickisch O, Seidler U, *et al.* Intravenous iron sucrose versus oral iron supplementation for the treatment of iron deficiency anemia in patients with inflammatory bowel disease - a randomized, controlled, open-label, multicenter study. *Am J Gastroenterol* 2005; 100(11): 2503-9.
21. Lindgren S, Wikman O, Befrits R, *et al.* Intravenous iron sucrose is superior to oral iron sulphate for correcting anaemia and restoring iron stores in IBD patients: a randomized, controlled, evaluator-blind, multicentre study. *Scand J Gastroenterol* 2009; 44: 838-45.
22. Semrin G, Fishman DS, Bousvaros A, *et al.* Impaired intestinal iron absorption in Crohn's disease correlates with disease activity and markers of inflammation. *Inflamm Bowel Dis* 2006; 12(12): 1101-6.
23. Gisbert JP, Bermejo F, Pajares R, *et al.* Oral and intravenous iron treatment in inflammatory bowel disease: hematological response and quality of life improvement. *Inflamm Bowel Dis* 2009; 15(10): 1485-91.
24. Kulnigg S, Stoinov S, Simanenkov V, *et al.* A novel intravenous iron formulation for treatment of anemia in inflammatory bowel disease: the ferric carboxymaltose (FERINJECT) randomized controlled trial. *Am J Gastroenterol* 2008; 103: 1182-92.
25. Evstatiev R, Marteau P, Iqbal T, *et al.* FERGIcor, a randomized controlled trial on ferric carboxymaltose for iron deficiency anemia in inflammatory bowel disease. *Gastroenterology* 2011; 141: 846-53.
26. Koutroubakis IE, Oustamanolakis P, Karakoidas C, *et al.* Safety and efficacy of total-dose infusion of low-molecular-weight iron dextran for iron deficiency anemia in patients with inflammatory bowel disease. *Dig Dis Sci* 2010; 55: 2327-31.
27. Gasche C, Waldhoer T, Feichtenschlager T, *et al.* Prediction of response to iron sucrose in inflammatory bowel disease-associated anemia. *Am J Gastroenterol* 2001; 96: 2382-7.
28. Pastrana RJ, Torres EA, Arroyo JM, *et al.* Iron-deficiency anemia as presentation of pouchitis. *J Clin Gastroenterol* 2007; 41: 41-4.

Chapter 21

Bone diseases in inflammatory bowel disease

Charlotte Pither BSc (Hons) BM MRCP Specialist Registrar, Department of Gastroenterology, University Hospital Southampton, Southampton, UK
J. R. Fraser Cummings FRCP DPhil Consultant Gastroenterologist, Department of Gastroenterology, University Hospital Southampton, Southampton, UK

Overview

Chronic inflammatory disorders such as inflammatory bowel disease (IBD) are associated with bone disease including osteoporosis, osteopenia and vitamin D deficiency [1].

Osteoporosis is a major public health problem and in the UK, is estimated to cause in excess of 200,000 fractures per year and is associated with considerable mortality of up to 30% at 1 year [2]. Osteoporosis costs the UK more than £1 billion a year [3].

Whilst osteoporosis is more common than vitamin D deficiency, in the UK, low vitamin D status is a frequent finding in the background population. Patients with IBD are at particular risk due to the inflammatory process, malabsorption and treatments.

The high incidence of metabolic bone disease in gastrointestinal diseases is well recognised; however, studies suggest screening and treatment can be sub-optimal [4]. UK guidelines on the management of osteoporosis have been available since 2007 [5], but there are no standardised guidelines for the management of vitamin D deficiency.

Introduction

The World Health Organisation (WHO) defines osteoporosis as a "systemic skeletal disease characterised by low bone mass and micro-architectural deterioration of bone tissue with a consequent increase in bone fragility and susceptibility to fracture" [6]. Risk factors for osteoporosis are shown in Table 1. Bone mineral density is the major determinant of bone strength which reaches a peak in the second to third decade after which it gradually declines. Women suffer from bone loss more rapidly than men and this is especially so in the postmenopausal years when 5-15% bone mass is lost in the first 5 years.

Bone remodelling is an active, progressive process and involves several cell populations, soluble mediators and receptors. Osteoporosis occurs if bone resorption exceeds bone formation. Reduced synthesis of bone matrix with normal bone resorption causes low turnover osteoporosis. High turnover osteoporosis is characterised by increased activity of osteoclasts and excessive resorption. Osteoporosis associated with inflammatory states tends to follow the high turnover pattern whereas corticosteroid-induced osteoporosis tends to follow the low turnover pattern.

Vitamin D homeostasis within the body is shown in Figure 1. It acts as a positive regulator in calcium and phosphate homeostasis as well as having a number of immune functions. It maintains serum calcium and phosphate ion concentrations at the levels needed for optimal neuromuscular activity and bone mineralisation. Intestinal absorption of calcium occurs mostly in the more proximal segments of the small bowel and is dependent on vitamin D-dependent Ca^{2+}-binding protein; calcium is also absorbed in the kidneys by both parathyroid hormone and vitamin D-stimulated mechanisms. Vitamin D is absorbed in the duodenum and jejunum. In Crohn's disease (CD), calcium and vitamin D absorption can be impaired by diseased small bowel or as a result of resection, resulting in muscle weakness and skeletal demineralisation.

Observational studies show that vitamin D insufficiency is widespread in many northern regions of the world including the UK. In humans, >90% of vitamin D is synthesised in the skin after exposure to ultraviolet radiation.

Table 1. Risk factors for osteoporosis in the general population and in IBD patients.

General risk factors for fracture related to low bone mineral density	Risk factors for osteoporosis in IBD [1, 10]
Increasing age	Increasing age
Previous fragility fracture	Previous fragility fracture
Medications: • Anticonvulsants • Proton pump inhibitors • Aromatase inhibitors • SSRI antidepressants • Methotrexate	Type of IBD – greater risk after ileal resection in Crohn's disease
Low physical activity level	Chronic inflammatory activity
Short fertile period in women	Chronic/recurrent steroid use
Family history of osteoporosis	Vitamin D insufficiency/deficiency
Smoking	Family history of osteoporosis
Low calcium intake	Smoking
Female gender	Female gender
Low body weight	Low body weight
Alcohol excess	Hypogonadism

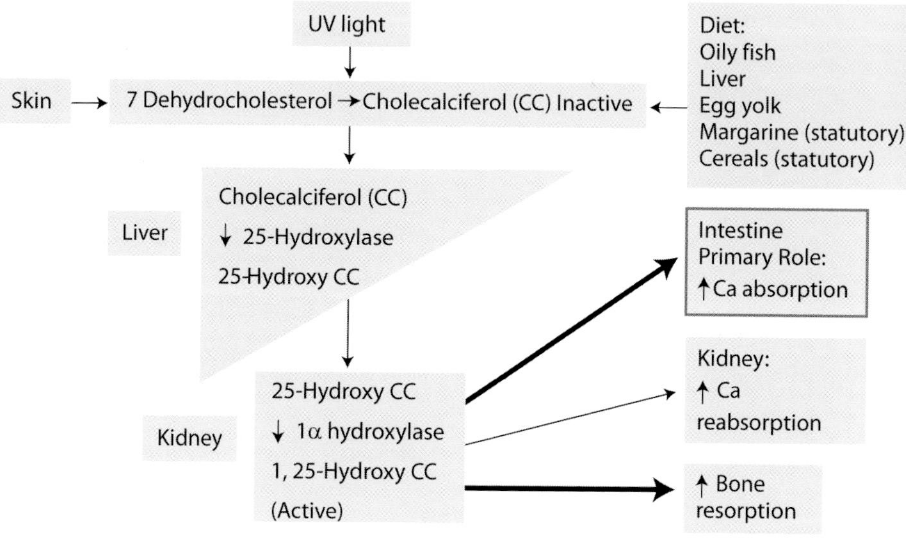

Figure 1. Vitamin D homeostasis.

In the UK for 6 months of the year, 90% of our landmass lies above the latitude where the wavelength of light is that which is required for vitamin D synthesis. Consequently, a large proportion of the population relies on dietary sources. A recent national survey showed >50% of the population have insufficient vitamin D status and 16% have severe deficiency during the winter and spring. The highest rates of deficiency are in the far north [7].

Serum total vitamin D levels offer an accurate reflection of status and definitions in widespread use are: >50ng/L normal; 25-50ng/L insufficiency; <25ng/L deficient.

Osteoporosis

Fracture is the only clinically important outcome of osteoporosis. For all fractures, the odds ratio is approximately 1.4 for CD and 1.2 for ulcerative colitis (UC). The risk appears slightly greater for hip fracture; the odds ratio is 1.86 for CD and 1.4 for UC [8]. The risk of vertebral fracture is underestimated as most studies rely on reporting of fractures; one study which screened patients with lumbar dual-energy X-ray absorptiometry (DXA) scans found a fracture prevalence of 22% [5], although our own data do not support this high figure (unpublished observation).

Risk factors for osteoporosis which apply to the general population apply equally to IBD patients, but there are other important factors which contribute to risk [1,5] (Table 1). The pathogenesis of osteoporosis in IBD is incompletely understood but there is evidence that inflammation *per se* is a major contributor to osteoporosis risk.

Physiology of bone turnover in chronic inflammatory states and with corticosteroid therapy

Physiology of bone turnover in chronic inflammatory states and with corticosteroid therapy is outlined in Figure 2. Osteoblasts are derived from multipotential mesenchymal cells that can differentiate into either marrow stromal cells or adipocytes [1]. The factors that signal the development of osteoblasts are not fully understood. Osteoclasts are multinucleated macrophage-like giant cells which resorb bone. They are haemopoietic in origin and derive from myeloid precursors that give rise to macrophages and dendritic cells. Signals that control osteoclasts to form and resorb bone involve several transcription factors and cytokines. Osteoclasts are highly motile and move across the bone surface and resorb large areas of bone.

Inflammation-related osteoporosis is driven by activation of osteoclasts and this cell type is of critical importance. In health, a neutral balance between osteoclastic and osteoblastic action exists. In inflammatory conditions, a soluble mediator, RANKL (a member of the TNF family) is produced by activated T lymphocytes. RANKL induces and activates

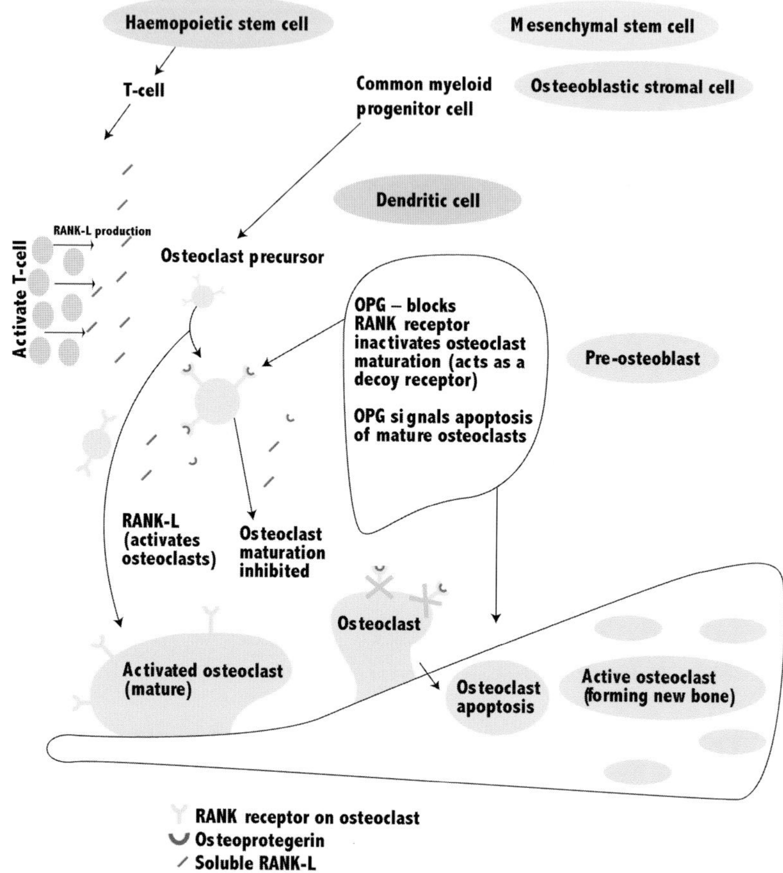

Figure 2. Bone loss in inflammatory states. In health there is a neutral balance between osteoclastic (bone breakdown) and osteoblastic action (bone formation). RANK-L which is produced by T-lymphocytes binds to the RANK receptors on the osteoclast precursor cells to turn them into mature active osteoclasts. OPG which is a natural decoy receptor has two specific actions: firstly, it blocks the RANK receptor and this stops maturation of the pre-osteoclasts; secondly, it signals for apoptosis of mature osteoclasts. In active inflammatory disease states, levels of activated T-cells are increased which results in increased RANK-L. If RANK-L overrules OPG, then osteoclasts survive beyond their normal life expectancy and the balance falls in favour of increased osteoclast action. Additionally, pro-inflammatory cytokines such as IL-1beta, IL-6 and TNF-alpha are in abdundance and promote osteoclastogenesis and bone resorption in synergy with RANK-L. IFN-gamma is also present promoting bone loss by increasing antigen presentation and T-cell activation.

osteoclasts and bone loss is promoted. Other pro-inflammatory cytokines such as IL-1β, IL-6 and TNFα also promote osteoclastogenesis too. Control of inflammation is therefore vitally important in minimising bone loss.

Corticosteriod therapy negatively affects bone mass by various mechanisms, including impairment of osteoblast function, reduction in intestinal calcuim absorption and increased renal calcuim excretion. Together this leads to a state of low turnover bone loss. There is some evidence to suggest that a higher daily dose of corticosteroids (rather than cumulative dose) poses a greater fracture risk, and at lower doses there appears to be only a minimal effect on bone formation, which may be explained by reduced inflammation offsetting the effects of corticosteroid [5]. Other studies suggest that the risk reverts to baseline once steroids are stopped [5].

Diagnostic tests

In the UK, dual-energy X-ray absorptiometry (DXA) is the most widely available and preferred method available to measure bone mineral density (BMD). It is non-invasive, accurate and a precise method of assessing BMD. Other diagnostic tests include ultrasound but this does not measure BMD which is the measure WHO currently uses to diagnose and define osteoporosis (Table 2). Another drawback is that ultrasound cannot be used to monitor response to treatment but it does provide an independent predictor of who will fracture [5]. Dual-photon absorptiometry (DPA) and quantitative computed tomography (pQCT) are less frequently used techniques.

Results of bone density scans are presented in three different ways:

- Bone mineral density (g/cm^2).
- Z-score: the number of standard deviations above or below the mean for the patient's age, sex and ethnicity.
- T-score: the number of standard deviations above or below the mean for a healthy 30-year-old adult of the same sex and ethnicity as the patient.

Table 2. The World Health Organization defined categories based on bone density in white women.	
Normal bone	T-score better than -1
Osteopenia	T-score between -1 and -2.5
Osteoporosis	T-score less than -2.5

BMD alone is a poor indicator of assessing fracture risk and therefore a DXA result needs to be interpreted following detailed assessment of risk factors (Table 1). The FRAX® tool [9] has been developed by WHO to evaluate fracture risk and is based on individual patient models which integrate the risk factors and associated clinical factors as well as bone mineral density (BMD) at the femoral neck. The FRAX® algorithms give the 10-year probability of both hip and major osteoporotic fracture. Major comorbidity is factored into the risk but there are no data looking at validity in IBD patients and it has not been validated in patients under 40 years old.

Screening

The purpose of screening is to detect the presence of osteoporosis in an individual who does not present with any symptoms of the disease with the purpose of taking measures to reduce fractures. The fact that IBD patients are at increased risk due to the factors previously outlined raises the question about who should be screened. BMD as a screening test should be used to inform specific actions or treatments. Some recommend selective screening once a thorough risk assessment has been undertaken [1, 10]. The American Gastroenterology Association (AGA) suggests that if one or more of the risk factors for osteoporosis in IBD are present, as listed in the second column of Table 1, patients should undergo initial screening with DXA which should be repeated at 2-3 years or, in the event of continued corticosteroid use, after 1 year. Alternatives include screening all patients but to justify this would need further evaluation of its cost-effectiveness or simply to treat all patients with calcium and vitamin D supplements.

Prevention

Achieve sustained steroid-free remission

Studies comparing patients in remission to those with active disease suggest that patients in remission have significantly higher Z-scores, and the Z-score correlates with duration of remission.

Patients on azathioprine have significantly increased Z-scores, possibly due to control of the inflammatory disease [1]. TNFα is believed to be pivotal in the pathogenesis of inflammation-associated osteoporosis and therefore it would be reasonable to assess whether anti-TNF therapies influence bone health. Some studies have shown increased markers of bone formation without any increase in bone resorption [11], but data on this are limited and more studies are needed.

General lifestyle measures

The impact of weight-bearing physical activity on the bone health of patients with IBD has not been investigated, but as the benefits of regular activity on muscle mass and bone mass in healthy subjects are clearly documented, then it would be reasonable to assume that this is the case with patients with IBD.

Calcium and vitamin D intake

Bone loss in patients who start treatment with steroids occurs rapidly, generally correlates with dose and can be severe in steroid-naïve patients. All patients with IBD on corticosteriods should receive calcium and vitamin D supplements. Calcium and vitamin D are effective for the prevention of postmenopausal osteoporosis but are not a treatment *per se* [1].

Avoid or minimise the use of corticosteroids

There are some acute situations when steroids are indicated, but avoiding or minimising the use of corticosteroids is advocated. Budesonide has been shown to have a beneficial effect on the prevention of early bone loss in corticosteroid-naïve CD patients [1], although its use may be limited by its efficacy and selective site of action in the gut. If steroids are needed, they should be given for the shortest time at the lowest effective dose. Bisphosphonates are currently recommended for those over 65 or who have had a fragility fracture if they are started on a course of steroids [5]. In those under 65, a risk assessment should be carried out and DXA performed in high-risk individuals and bisphosphonates started if the T-score <-1.5.

Treatment of osteoporosis (Figure 3)

Many of the studies evaluating different treatments have been conducted in large populations of postmenopausal women and therefore treatment recommendations are based on that data with the assumption in many cases that it can be extrapolated to the IBD population.

Calcium and vitamin D

Adequate intake is important and is normally supplemented orally. In patients with a short bowel, parenteral vitamin D may be necessary although this tends to be poorly absorbed.

Bisphosphonates

These are pyrophosphate analogues and work by inhibiting osteoclast action. There is overall good evidence for their efficacy in treating patients with low impact fractures or a T-score of <-2.5. Patients with a short bowel may require parenteral bisphosphonates due to insufficient absorption of the oral preparation and there are now several preparations available including a yearly infusion.

Other treatments

Calcitonin and strontium ranelate are alternative treatments available for specific circumstances. Hormone replacement therapy use is associated with a significant reduction in fracture rates [1] and used to be a major treatment modality in postmenopausal osteoporosis until 2002 when a possible link with ischaemic heart disease and breast cancer was identified.

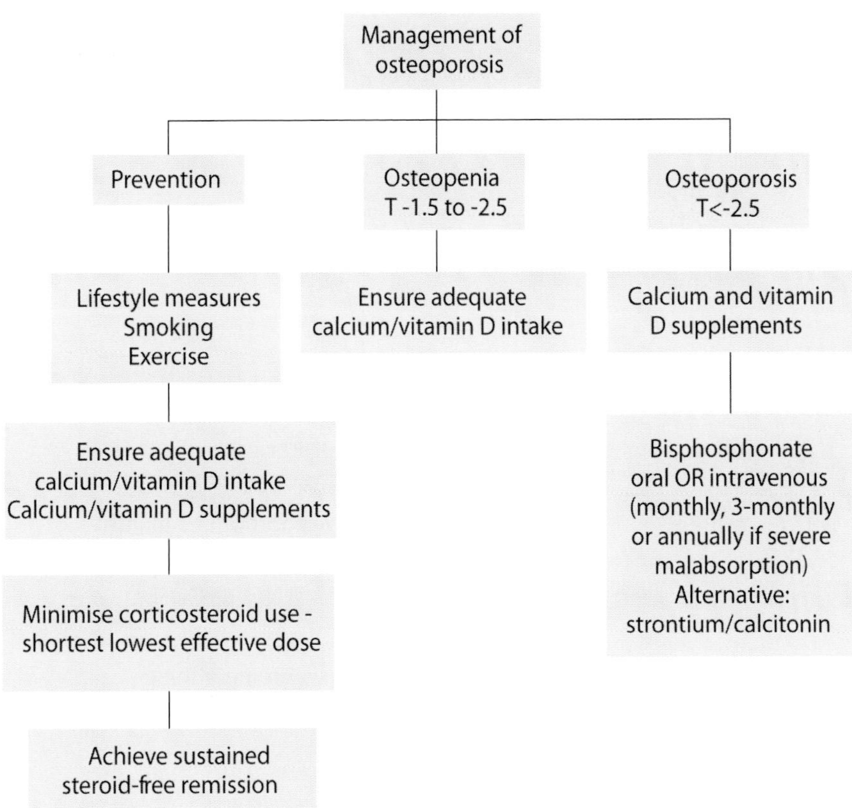

Figure 3. Algorithm for the management of osteoporosis.

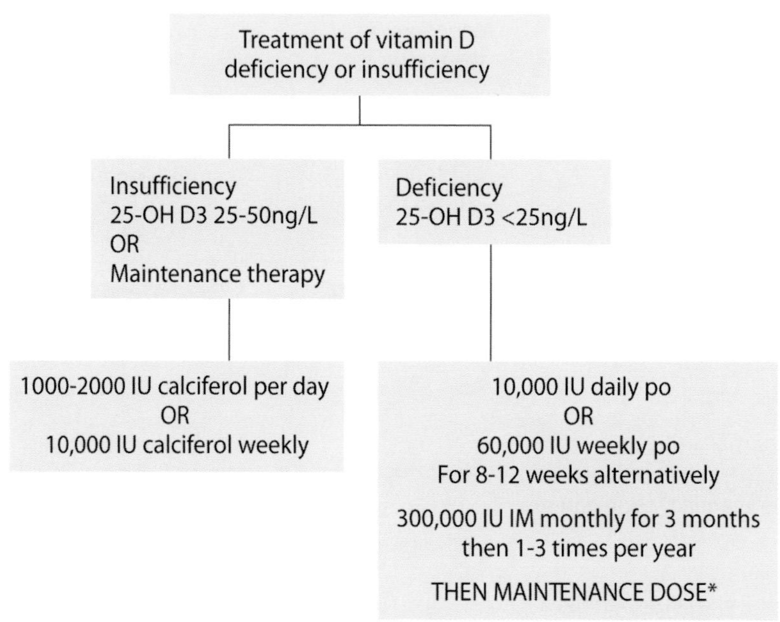

*In those with malabsorption or short bowel syndrome, a three-monthly intramuscular injection of 300,000 IU may be given.

Figure 4. Suggested treatment algorithm for vitamin D deficiency [7].

Vitamin D deficiency and insufficiency

Osteomalacia is the manifestation of profound vitamin D deficiency in adults and is preventable. Symptoms of vitamin D deficiency can be vague and often attributed to other factors: they include muscle weakness, generalised muscle aches and pains, proximal weakness and bone pain, particularly in the ribs and hips. The alkaline phosphatase and parathyroid hormone levels may be raised in about 80% of cases of osteomalacia and occasionally hypocalcaemia and hypophosphataemia may be present. Low bone mineral density on DXA or osteopenia on X-ray should trigger assessment of vitamin D status.

There is a high prevalence of vitamin D deficiency in the background population [8] and with the additional risks attributed to IBD, there is a rationale that all patients with IBD should have their vitamin D and parathyroid hormone (PTH) levels checked at regular intervals, although there are no standardised guidelines at present.

A suggested treatment algorithm for confirmed deficiency is shown in Figure 4. It should be noted that practice varies considerably. As few patients have a reversible aetiology, treatment should be long-term. Abnormalities of PTH and alkaline phosphatase can take up to 3 months to improve and up to a year to normalise. Poor compliance in the longer term with calcium/vitamin D supplements can arise as the calcium component makes the preparation unpalatable. Compliance with calciferol alone is better [8] and the calcium component rarely needed. There are no national guidelines for monitoring response to therapy but the authors suggest 6-monthly assessment of vitamin D levels would be appropriate in most cases.

Conclusions

Patients with inflammatory bowel disease are at significantly increased risk of metabolic bone diseases. Both osteoporosis and vitamin D deficiency are long-term complications which are potentially preventable and treatable. Evidence shows screening for these problems is often overlooked in the clinic setting. The importance of screening in order to take preventative measures followed by timely appropriate management cannot be over-emphasized and forms an important component of providing high quality care to patients with inflammatory bowel disease.

Key points

- **The need for osteoporosis screening should be considered in every IBD patient.**
- **Co-prescribe calcium and vitamin D with corticosteroids.**
- **Vitamin D deficency is common in IBD patients and often overlooked.**
- **Sustained steriod-free remission is key to the prevention of bone disease.**

References

1. Tilg, H, Moschen AR, Kaser A, *et al.* Gut inflammation and osteoporosis: basic and clinical concepts. *Gut* 2008; 57: 684-94.
2. Guidelines development group Royal College of Physicians. Osteoporosis: clinical guidelines for prevention and treatment. London: RCP, 1999.
3. Cooper C, Atkinson EJ, Jacobsen SJ, *et al.* Population-based study of the survival after osteoporotic fractures. *Am J Epid* 1993; 137: 1001-5.
4. Reddy SI, Friedman S, Telford J, *et al.* Are patients with IBD receiving optimal care? *Am J Gastroenterology* 2005; 100: 1357-61.
5. Lewis NR, Scott BB. Guidelines for Osteoporosis in IBD and Coeliac Disease. British Society of Gastroenterology, 2007.
6. World Health Organisation (WHO). Assessment of fracture risk and its application to screening for post-menopausal osteoporosis. Report of a WHO study group. *WHO Tech Series* 1994; 843: 1-129.
7. Pear A, Cheetham T. Diagnosis and management of vitamin D deficiency. *BMJ Clinical Review* 2010; 340: b5664.
8. San Staa, Cooper C, Brusse L, *et al.* Inflammatory bowel disease and the risk of fracture. *Gastroenterology* 2003; 125: 1592-7.
9. FRAX and the assessment of fracture risk in men and women in the UK. *Osteoporosis International* 2008; 19: 385-97.
10. Bernstein C, leslie WD, Leboff M. AGA technical review on osteoporosis in gastrointestinal diseased. *Gastroenterology* 2003; 123: 795-841.
11. Abreu MT, Geller J, Vasiliauska E, *et al.* Treatment with infliximab is associated with increased markers of bone formation in patients with Crohn's disease. *J Clin Gastr* 2006; 40: 55-63.